MINDFUL
DRINKING

HOW CUTTING
DOWN CAN CHANGE
YOUR LIFE

ROSAMUND DEAN

D1637686

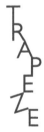

First published in Great Britain in 2017 by Trapeze,
an imprint of The Orion Publishing Group Ltd
This paperback edition published in 2020 by Trapeze,
Carmelite House, 50 Victoria Embankment,
London EC4Y 0DZ

An Hachette UK company

1 3 5 7 9 10 8 6 4 2

Copyright © Rosamund Dean 2017

The moral right of Rosamund Dean to be identified as
the author of this work has been asserted in accordance with
the Copyright, Designs and Patents Act of 1988.

All rights reserved. No part of this publication may be
reproduced, stored in a retrieval system, or transmitted
in any form or by any means, electronic, mechanical,
photocopying, recording, or otherwise, without the
prior permission of both the copyright owner and the
above publisher of this book.

A CIP catalogue record for this book is
available from the British Library.

ISBN (Paperback) 978 1409 1 8489 8

Typeset by Input Data Services Ltd, Somerset

Printed and bound in Great Britain by Clays Ltd, Elcograf S.p.A.

Every effort has been made to ensure that the information in the book is accurate. The
information in this book may not be applicable in each individual case so it is advised that
professional medical advice is obtained for specific health matters and before changing any
medication or dosage. Neither the publisher nor author accepts any legal responsibility for any
personal injury or other damage or loss arising from the use of the information in this book. In
addition if you are concerned about your diet or exercise regime and wish to change them, you
should consult a health practitioner first.

MIX
Paper from
responsible sources
FSC® C104740

www.orionbooks.co.uk

For Jonathan

INTRODUCTION

Ever woken up with the queasy sense of paranoia that you said the wrong thing to the wrong person at work drinks the night before? Ever felt that it seemed unsociable not to get drunk at a friend's birthday? Ever had a hangover that only a Bloody Mary with brunch could cure? Ever been annoyed with yourself for polishing off the entire bottle of wine when you only intended to have one glass with dinner?

If that sounds familiar (and it did to me), you probably already know that you ought to cut back on your alcohol consumption. But at the same time, you probably don't really want to. Drinking is fun, celebratory and enhances confidence on your good days, as much as it relieves stress on your bad days. We are societally programmed to drink, thanks to the ubiquity of alcohol in music, film and television, not to mention on our Facebook and Instagram feeds. Our family gatherings wouldn't feel right without wine, and our urban families are built on booze. Whether bonding with colleagues, a new partner or 'mum friends', it almost always involves alcohol.

You might believe, like I did, that non-drinkers are smug and boring. Even words that mean not drinking – such as 'sober' and 'dry' – have alternative meanings of 'humourless' and 'dull'. And soft drinks sound considerably less fun than hard. Am I right?

As a tobacco lobbyist announces in the satirical film *Thank You For Smoking*: 'Cigarettes are cool, available and addictive. The job is almost done for us.' You could say the same about alcohol. Except, unlike smoking, drinking is not only socially acceptable, but socially *expected*.

Of course, there is a dark side to this. As a causal factor in more than 60 medical conditions – including not only the obvious ones such as liver disease but also everything from depression to cancer – alcohol now costs the National Health Service £3.5 billion per year.[1] That's £120 for every single tax payer. Perhaps surprisingly, it's the higher-tax payers that cause the most problems. Alcohol consumption increases alongside wealth, with almost one in five people earning over £40,000 per year drinking alcohol at least five days a week, and being more likely to 'binge' on their heaviest drinking day.[2] (Oh, and binge-drinking means consuming anything over three pints of beer or two large glasses of wine in one sitting. Yep, really.) If the medical stats don't hit a

1 Alcohol Concern
2 Office for National Statistics

2

nerve, allow me to appeal to your vanity. A large glass of wine contains as many calories as a chocolate bar, and the added sugar in alcoholic drinks is breaking down the collagen in our skin, causing wrinkles and sagging. Aside from the effects on our bodies and skin, I think you already know that you'd be a better colleague, partner, friend or parent without that hangover. Undeterred, British people drank 40 million litres of prosecco in 2016. With alcohol, sugar and carbonation constituting the hat-trick of dentistry's worst nightmares, it's enough to make all your teeth fall out in protest.

But I'm not just here to throw terrifying stats at you. I'm here to help.

There are a million books out there about cutting alcohol out of your life completely – but this isn't one of them. Most people don't want to do that. I certainly don't. Who wants to attend a wedding, birthday party or – God forbid – a date when stone-cold sober? I love the fizz of the bubbles in champagne when toasting a friend's celebration, or the kick of an ice-cold gin and tonic on a hot day. In today's all-or-nothing culture, where everyone is either a prosecco-gulping, devil-may-care hedonist or a joyless, clean-eating teetotaller, people seem to have forgotten that there is a middle ground.

And that's what this book is all about. The advice here is not intended for people with a serious drinking problem, or a physical dependency on alcohol. (By that I mean people who crave alcohol at any time of day and have become secretive or dishonest about their drinking.) For those with a severe alcohol addiction, many experts believe complete abstinence may be the only answer. Rather, this book is intended for the vast majority of us who are not alcoholics but are aware that we drink more than is healthy and want to break out of that cycle to find a middle ground. Our dependence on alcohol is less an addiction, more a habit. So while we don't want to give up drinking altogether, we do want to wake up clear-headed because we were able to resist that third glass of wine the night before.

Moderation might sound deceptively simple, but it's really far more complicated than abstinence. You might decide not to drink too much at that work event or friend's party, but after one or two drinks your willpower and decision-making skills tend to go out of the window. Making a lasting change is particularly challenging, since moderation requires constant awareness of your behaviour and decisions.

One of the most common reasons for drinking too much is doing so without really thinking about it. Accepting a glass of wine because everyone else is having one, or pouring yourself a drink at home every night, purely out of habit. Mindlessly doing something because you've always done it is a tough habit to break, but it can be done. It's going to involve clearing your head and paying conscious attention to your thoughts and behaviour.

So how do we break those habits and start to drink with full awareness and responsibility? Mindful drinking is exactly what it sounds like: it's the opposite of drinking without thinking. Mindfulness has had a lot of press in recent years, and if you're anything like me you've probably tried meditation, and given up on it. The benefits of meditation are extremely seductive: reduced stress, improved concentration, more productivity and the ability to make better decisions. But I struggled to find the time (or, indeed, the patience) to make meditation a regular practice.

However, I've now learned that you don't have to sit in the lotus position for twenty minutes every day to bring mindfulness into your life, and I'm going to show you how incorporating mindful awareness into your everyday activities will make your journey to moderating your drinking not only easier, but something that will come naturally.

If you need reminding as to why you should approach your drinking mindfully, here are a few convincing arguments. Moderating your drinking will improve your mood, your digestion, your skin and your body, as well as sharpen your brain. Everything from your bank balance to your sex life will improve. It also automatically moderates other bad habits, such as social smoking, hungover binge-eating and mainlining coffee to get through the day after a night of fitful drunk sleep. We live in tense times, where people see alcohol as a stress-buster but, actually, the link between excessive alcohol and anxiety is inescapable.

By bringing mindfulness into your life, not only will you reap the benefits of having a more moderate relationship with alcohol, you will also improve your concentration and decisiveness, giving you a stronger sense of empathy and making self-control in other areas of your life a breeze.

At first glance I might seem an unlikely advocate of moderate drinking. I spent my teenage years in a beery haze in the ladette era of the 1990s, and my twenties downing cheap white wine as a keen young journalist. I have vomited on tube platforms and out of taxi windows. I have done more than my fair share of drunk texting and ill-advised rants at the office Christmas party. At my regular book group, it was compulsory to arrive armed with two bottles of prosecco each, and we always got through the whole lot.

Waking up after my thirtieth birthday, I realised that my lifestyle was beginning to impact on my body, mind, skin and career. I had friends who hit their thirties and became health freaks, cutting out alcohol entirely, but that felt extreme to me – I had never been arrested for drunken behaviour, or lost a job or destroyed a relationship because of booze, nor had any kind of rock-bottom moment. As I wailed to the health director on the women's magazine where I worked (she sat beside me, so she experienced the hangovers and the post-carby-lunch crashes more than anyone): 'I don't want to give up alcohol completely. I just want to drink a bit less.'

Eventually, she asked me to write about it, sending me off to a Harley Street psychologist and hypnotherapist to learn how to control my drinking. The programme wasn't about giving up; it was simply about having control and learning how to be moderate. A few hypnotherapy sessions didn't quite change my life overnight (our health director raised an eyebrow when I proudly told her I *only* had five glasses of fizz at that month's book group), but it sparked a fascination with the social, behavioural and psychological reasons as to why we over-drink.

When I was pregnant with my son, I found it easy to not drink. 'I'm pregnant' is one of the few failsafe reasons you can give in any social situation that won't lead to people trying to pressure you into drinking (other than 'I'm driving'). And I believe the odd drink in pregnancy is fine, so I still had champagne on special occasions, or wine with a meal. At the time, I was so delighted with how easy it had been to cut down that I was sure I would stick with moderate drinking for life. After this baby is born, my tolerance will be low from nine months of hardly drinking, I thought. I'll be tired, due to having a new baby, I'll be on maternity leave, so work events won't be a problem for a while, and I'll also have baby weight to lose. I believed that this perfect storm of elements would naturally change my drinking habits forever. Looking back, it's hilarious how naive I was. Within minutes of getting home from hospital, my husband and I were drinking champagne. I mean, how could we not? We had something to celebrate. (I should add that my husband was so tired when he bought the champagne, he failed to notice they hadn't removed the security tag. He had to go back to the shop to have them take it off before we could open it. Yes, this was our priority as soon as we got our baby home.)

Like many people, I took my local NCT (National Childbirth Trust) ante-natal sessions to find a group of local 'mum friends' to hang out with while on maternity leave. NCT classes are a lottery and not everyone has a great experience, but I hit the jackpot with a bunch of cool, funny, interesting women who, I was delighted to find, never turned up for lunch without a bottle. I would always take a glass of wine into baby cinema rather than a coffee because, why the hell not? If my son Ezra was grumpy because of teething or reflux, my husband would bring home a 'gin in a tin' to say well done for getting through the day. And we'd always have wine with dinner, because I wasn't pregnant any more so it felt like a novelty to be drinking together again. When I went out in the evening, to see friends or work colleagues or my book group, I felt that drinking was a way to show them that I hadn't changed. I might be a mum now, guys, but I'm still fun! I soon realised I was drinking just as much, if not more, than ever. The difference was, I could no longer sleep it off, and it was showing, in my skin and body. (I'll never forget being asked when my baby was due, ten months after he was born.)

Of course, my slide back into heavy drinking within weeks after giving birth was down to me, and was in no way attributable to my friends, husband, NCT gang, book group, colleagues or anyone else. I should have been able to say no to that second or third drink. But the problem was, as a successful, determined person in other parts of my life, I believed that I could simply use willpower to continue to drink moderately after pregnancy.

So I didn't set myself goals or make a plan or give it any other thought than, I'll just drink less from now on. I thought my rational brain would make those decisions, without realising that's not how it works at all.

Writing this book has been a journey for me because it was through the extensive research and interviews with psychologists and behaviour-change experts that I realised why I hadn't been able to cut down in the past, despite wanting to do so. Having a baby changed my attitude towards drinking, and hypnosis took me some way towards changing my behaviour, but, ultimately, they both failed because I failed to commit to a plan for life. And you *do* need a plan, because this isn't something that's going to happen with no effort on your part. It's why so many people fall off the wagon after successfully completing Dry January. They don't have a plan for the rest of the year, so they slip back into learned behaviours.

I decided to write this book because I was determined to change my relationship with drinking for the long term, and share what I had learned with others who are in the same boat. I wanted to put myself in control, rather than allowing alcohol to control me. Over the course of my research, I started changing my habits. I realised that I needed to understand the real reasons why I drank too much, and be able to identify my triggers. I worked out a plan to adopt a more moderate approach to drinking, and a way to stick to it. I learnt to be more mindful in my day-to-day life and, as a result, I can now see the underlying issues when I want a drink, and I am able to be less judgemental of myself if I slip up (which is inevitable, by the way). The old me could never have imagined that I would become that person who happily gets tipsy at a wedding but isn't hung-over the next day. The person who enjoys one glass of wine with dinner but doesn't need a whole bottle. The person who has several alcohol-free days every week without it being a struggle or feeling like a deprivation. And I'm going to show you how you can be that person, too.

Over the course of this book, I will take you through The Problem: the reasons why we over-drink and why it is such a pervading issue in our society. I will give you The Incentive: the health and wellbeing benefits that will inspire you to make this positive change. I'll explain the practice of mindfulness and the ways in which it will help you develop a more moderate attitude towards drinking. And then we'll get to The Plan: a four-point method to change your drinking habits for life. Using the four Ms: Measure, Monitor, Manage and Maintain, you will assess how much you drink, monitor bad habits and triggers, and take a clean break – which means going alcohol-free for 28 days. Don't be apprehensive about this part of the process, it's vital to identify your danger zones, and I'll provide plenty of advice and tips for surviving it. The final hurdle (actually a bad analogy, because this is a marathon, not a sprint) is reintroducing alcohol into your life in a more moderate way. Managing your behaviour and maintaining a moderate relationship with drinking, by establishing habits and techniques to make your new lifestyle stick, as well as dealing with slip-ups in a positive way.

This book will give you conscious tools to help you deal with every stumbling block, from pushily boozy friends to non-drunk dating, combining my own personal experience with advice from behaviour-change experts, psychologists and successful moderate drinkers to convey the latest research and practical advice. You will finish this book feeling motivated and empowered to change your relationship with alcohol forever.

1

THE PROBLEM

Before you start this journey, it's important for you to understand your own personal reasons why you drink too much, because you can't fix something if you don't know why it's broken. In this chapter, I'm going to take you through the cultural and societal reasons as to why we over-drink, identify the personality types that are more prone to do so, and the role of stress and anxiety in your drinking habits.

To solve a problem, you must first acknowledge it, but most of us don't like to think of ourselves as having a 'problem' with drinking. We often joke that we're 'addicted' to cheese/Instagram/*Love Island*, but we would never describe our alcohol use in those terms, even though we often drink more than we want to or intend to. You might reassure yourself that you don't have a physical dependency on alcohol. It isn't damaging your relationships or career. You're not gulping straight vodka from that water bottle on your desk all day. So what's the problem? Well, I used to think the same thing. Until I realised that daily drinking, while not affecting my life in any dramatic way, was slowly and increasingly less subtly disrupting everything from my skin to my mood, all while storing up health problems for the future. So, yes, you might not have A Problem, but it certainly is a lower-case problem. The fact that you have picked up this book means that you know you need to do something about it.

Regret and self-judgement will keep you in the vicious circle of drinking too much and feeling bad about it, so I want you to understand that being sucked into this heavy-drinking culture is not your fault. Repeat after me: it is not your fault. Say it again, like Robin Williams in *Good Will Hunting*. It is *not* your fault. Your drinking is the result of a lifetime of psychological conditioning. Your brain can't be blamed for forging neural pathways that believe drinking is vital for everything from celebration to stress relief to socialising. That's just the world in which we grew up.

Your friends and family, work colleagues, advertisements, social media . . . so much of our environment is steeped in booze. The fact that drinking is such a part of celebratory social occasions is a triumph of marketing. We all like to think we're immune from the tricks of advertising, but it insidiously infiltrates our subconscious, making positive connections with alcohol, without our logical mind even realising it.

There is this perception that there are alcoholics, for whom sobriety is the only option, and then there are 'normal' drinkers, who drink because they like it. There is nothing in between. But I believe that everybody who drinks reasonably heavily, and reasonably regularly, has a certain degree of dependence on alcohol. That sounds terrifying, but acknowledging it is the first step towards changing your drinking. It was a revelation for me to realise that change wasn't going to happen on its own. I had to go through a process, and you can, too.

First of all, let's break down why it's so difficult.

THE EMOTIONAL PULL OF ALCOHOL

The trouble with drinking being so ingrained in our culture is that, even though you rationally know you need to drink less, you can't change your conscious mind without first changing your unconscious mind. No matter how logical a thought ('I should drink less because it's bad for my health'), your unconscious mind has formed long-standing beliefs that contradict that thought ('I need wine to have fun'). Your unconscious mind ignores rational reasoning because it's led by emotion, and your behaviour often follows on from that. You see the issue here?

Since alcohol is a key part of birthday parties, weddings and any occasion when there is anything to celebrate, our unconscious mind can be forgiven for creating hugely positive associations with it. If your work, social life and relationships are going well, you might even subconsciously credit alcohol with some of the success. After all, it was over drinks that you bonded with your friends, partner and colleagues. The truth is, you didn't *need* alcohol for any of that and, once you realise this, you will feel empowered to be able to enjoy a drink without any of the emotional baggage behind it, or having to immediately pour yourself another one.

My own drinking journey started long before I was even aware of it. Like most middle-class British people, I grew up in a house full of alcohol, laughter and friends. My parents embraced the idea of wine with every meal, and children being allowed a sip from a young age, as a sensibly sophisticated European approach. I couldn't remember at what age I had my first alcoholic drink, so I texted my mum to ask. The reply came back: 'a little wine, very occasionally, when you were ten-ish?' Part of me looks at my three-year-old boy and thinks giving a ten-year-old an alcoholic drink is recklessly irresponsible. But the rates of risky drinking in European countries where the family drinks together would seem to support my parents' choice. Italy, France and Spain were rated 'least risky' in World Health Organization data, which monitors things like daily drinking and binge-drinking,[3] working on a scale of one to five with five being most risky (Russia) and three being medium-risky (the UK). However, in those low-risk European countries where everybody has a healthy attitude towards moderate drinking, perhaps having sips of wine from a young

3 World Health Organization, Global Health Observatory, patterns of drinking score, 2014

age is fine. But in the UK, where pub culture takes the place of European-style café culture, and the effects of binge-drinking can be seen on high streets up and down the country, it makes less sense. Perhaps drinking at home with my family normalised something of which I should have been wary. It took me a long time to acknowledge that I needed to cut down, because I couldn't imagine a world in which I didn't have wine with dinner.

When young people initially don't like alcoholic drinks, we tend to tell them that it's an acquired taste, implanting in their minds that it's something grown-up and refined, like chilli olives or briney oysters, something that they should aspire to like. Realising this made me look at my own parenting behaviour. When my son makes a grab for my gin and tonic, assuming it's a fizzy water that he can have a swig of, I automatically say, 'Ezra, no, this is a grown-up drink.' At just three years old, he is learning that alcohol is for grown-ups, which means it's sophisticated and out-of-reach. I mean, I couldn't be making it any more attractive to him than if I shared a G&T with Spider-Man. A 2017 report by the Institute of Alcohol Studies found that even moderate drinking by parents has a negative effect on their offspring.[4] The children interviewed in the report were at best embarrassed and at worst worried about their parents' drinking. It makes for sobering reading.

4 Like Sugar For Adults: The effect of non-dependent parental drinking on children and families

Anyway, no matter how sensible the attitude towards drinking is in the home, it doesn't help that the larger cultural representation of alcohol is fun and aspirational. I was a teenager in the late 1990s, when the magazines I read were full of pictures of Britpop stars downing pints and tales of Kate Moss and Johnny Depp filling their bath with champagne. Sweet and cheap alcopops such as Hooch, WKD and Smirnoff Ice, clearly aimed at the younger drinker, saturated the market. Meanwhile, the 'ladette' was at her zenith. Here was Zoe Ball slurping from a bottle of Jack Daniels in Ibiza, there was Sara Cox stumbling out of the Met Bar. These riotously mouthy, booze-fuelled women gave zero fucks if you thought they were ladylike. It was a feminist movement, of a sort, celebrating the idea that women were just as capable of being raucous and leery as men. And it was empowering, in a way. In a Girl Power kind of way.

By 16 years old I was pulling on my Spice Girls-style mini dress and Buffalo boots and going to bars and clubs with friends every weekend (girls don't even need fake ID, it turns out). At university, with my halls of residence right next to the student union, I was pretty much drunk for three years. By the time I got my first job on a women's magazine when I was 21, I was already a hardened drinker with a high level of tolerance for the free booze constantly handed to me at press screenings, launches and events, proud of being able to drink the boys from the lads' mag in the next office under the table. I would turn up to work unsure whether I felt spaced out because of lack of sleep or if I was still a bit drunk. This pretty much carried on for over a decade, even if the drinking graduated from cheap white wine to a decent red, and from raucous nights out to dinner parties and – after having children – our sofa.

You get the picture: I was drunk for a long time, from a young age. So why did it take me so long to realise that I should do something about it? Well, I knew I wasn't an alcoholic. And one of the difficulties with moderation is that, while there are organisations like Alcoholics Anonymous that might work for those who want to concede defeat to their addiction and become teetotal, there has been nothing for those of us who just want to cut down.

Club Soda, however, could be our saviour. It's a UK-based movement to support people who want to cut down their drinking, stop for a bit, or quit. Co-founder Laura Willoughby MBE gave up drinking five years ago. 'I went through lots of attempts to moderate, but giving up is what worked for me,' she says. 'My off-switch broke at some point when I was about 36. But I realised, once I gave up, that one of the reasons I failed to moderate was because there wasn't anywhere for me to go. I wanted to create something to support people to do a self-guided journey, whatever their goal is. Something like Weight Watchers, but for booze.'

Her co-founder, Dr Jussi Tolvi, is a moderate drinker who laments how drinking is so interwoven in our society. 'When you say, "let's go for a drink", it only ever means one kind of drink,' he sighs. 'It's never a coffee.'

'So we've got all that cultural baggage to deal with alongside the fact that alcohol has altered our brains,' says Willoughby. 'There's the psychological impact of the fact that we have associated drinking with nearly every single element of the day – from getting home and relaxing to cooking to dealing with stress to "mummy time" . . . Our brains are all changed by the experiences that we have, and our experiences make up who we are. And so if all of your experiences have involved alcohol, and every way you have dealt with experiences has involved alcohol, then you really have to go through a process of unpicking that.'

I was the person who was always up for a drink. Whenever a friend would say, 'I'm not drinking tonight because I've got an early meeting,' or the other person at my work lunch said, 'I'll stick with water, thanks,' I would inwardly breathe a sigh of relief, because if that person was drinking, then damn right I was, too. I hated the idea of being the killjoy. Always being up for a drink was part of who I was. I love good food, I love parties, I love dancing, I even love karaoke. How could I still be that person who loves those things without drinking?

Gretchen Rubin is an American writer who studies habits and human nature, and her book *The Four Tendencies* is a clever guide to improving your life by knowing yourself better. I Skyped her in New York to get her take on my identity crisis. 'Often, for habits to change, an identity has to change, and that can be painful,' she told me. 'Whether you're the life of the party, who is always buying another round, or you're this cutting-edge person who is always up late, partying hard, it can be painful to let that go. But you have to let your identity evolve. Work out what it means to be the kind of person who's drinking in a different way. If you've spent your whole life despising those people, then it's hard now to become one of them.'

She's hit the nail on the head. I spent many years dismissing non-drinkers as smug and boring. To change my behaviour, I had to change my attitude, and that attitude was a big part of my identity. But I liked how Rubin described it as 'evolving' rather than being an abrupt change. We all grow and evolve; that's human nature. And if it stops me using my identity to keep me trapped in a series of unhealthy choices, that can only be a good thing. Realising that this was going to involve putting myself in situations where I would normally have a big glass of wine in my hand like a comfort blanket was hard. But I knew I had to reinvent myself and, once I'd decided that was what I was going to do, it became quite exciting. Who doesn't love a reinvention? It's a refresh, a reboot, a chance to reevaluate every aspect of your life.

Once you decide to frame it like this, it will help you realise that you have the power to control your drinking, and you can do so without feeling deprived or that you're sacrificing an important part of your identity. Rather, you're evolving in a positive way.

But this book is not about demonising drink. It's important

to acknowledge that a big part of the reason you drink is simply because you like it. Not only the taste, but also the ceremony of pouring a glass of red wine alongside a delicious meal, the anticipation of the pop of a champagne cork, or the memory of drinking cold foreign beer with handfuls of salty crisps on holiday with someone you love. The reasons why you enjoy drinking will still be there if you try to push them away, so instead embrace them. Think about them fully.

Learning to drink more moderately will mean that you can save your drinking occasions for those times when you will really enjoy it, rather than mindlessly throwing back cheap white wine at a work event or necking two G&Ts while struggling to put the children to bed.

Being unable to stop yourself after one or two drinks is not something you struggle with simply because you don't have much willpower, although I'm sure you have beaten yourself up over that in the past. In my experience, it is often the smartest, most successful and most strong-willed people that become stuck in a bad relationship with alcohol. This could be part of the reason why it's the highest-earning third of the population that drink the most. And could it be even worse if you're a woman?

ALCOHOL AND WOMEN

Women are drinking more than ever, whether we're throwing ourselves into work, with client dinners and colleague drinks as a vital part of that, or compulsively reaching for the wine as soon as the kids are in bed. A global study in 2016 showed that women are drinking as much as men – in many cases even more – for the first time in history.[5] Call it the post-*Sex and the City* effect, but women's personal relationships now revolve much more around wine or cocktails than they did even just 30 years ago.

A study by the Organisation for Economic Co-operation and Development showed British women are twice as likely to become problem drinkers if they've been to university.[6] The link between higher education and heavier drinking, suggests the report, is because professional women going into traditionally male-orientated careers such as finance feel that they have to 'keep up' with the men. It's also a way of managing stress levels, particularly if they're dealing with lack of salary parity and casual sexism in the workplace.

However, it is not only professional women who are drinking too much. Hypnotherapist Georgia Foster, founder of The

5 Study by the National Drug and Alcohol Research Centre of the University of New South Wales, Australia, published in the journal *BMJ Open*

6 *Tackling Harmful Alcohol Use*, published 2015

Drink Less Mind programme, says the majority of her clients are women in their thirties and forties, and it's a mix of women who are focused on their careers and stay-at-home mums. 'Drinking at home can often be triggered by loneliness,' she says. 'So it can happen if they're thinking, "I haven't got to where I wanted to be in life, I haven't met the man, I haven't had the kids." And, since boredom is another big trigger, a lot of mums will drink because they are stuck at home. It doesn't mean they don't want to be a parent, but their life is suddenly much more restrictive, so they have what I call "solo parties". When you're in your own environment, there's nobody watching and you don't have to drive anywhere, that glass of wine tends to go to two, then three, then the bottle's gone and you open a second bottle. That can be a very slippery slope.'

If you have kids you have probably already realised that, no matter how egalitarian your relationship with your partner, much of the caring and cleaning and organising and general drudgery of parenthood tends to fall to the mother. This is true at least in the early days when you're on maternity leave, and often in the long term, if you change your career or working hours to fit in around family life. That change can be incredibly discombobulating, and difficult to acknowledge, because women often feel they don't really have a right to be dissatisfied if they've been lucky enough to have children. Instead, they open another bottle.

Women now buy eight out of ten bottles of the wine that is

drunk at home in the UK,[7] and in the US, a recent report showed that high-risk drinking in women has surged by 58 per cent in ten years.[8] The alcohol industry has cottoned on to the fact that women are a key market and now spends a fortune marketing drinks directly to us. Much of this is done in a patronisingly unfeminist way, which is easy to ignore (pink Jack Daniel's with rose petals, anyone? Anyone?). But a lot of it is more insidious than that. From Baileys sponsoring the Women's Prize for Fiction, to phrases like 'mummy juice' and a beer brewed for chic athleticwear brand lululemon called Courageous Blonde. Scrolling through Instagram, I regularly see quotes such as: 'Motherhood has taught me that you don't need fun to have alcohol,' or 'Technically it's not drinking alone if your kids are home,' or 'Two or three glasses of wine a day can reduce your risk of giving a shit.' You've probably liked a quote like that in the past. You might even have posted one. And this is one of many ways in which alcohol becomes deeply embedded within our sense of identity.

7 *Women and Wine Survey* by Vinexpo, 2009
8 Research published in *JAMA Psychiatry*, 2017

WORKING OUT WHY YOU DRINK

The trouble with alcohol being so ingrained in our culture is that we often don't even realise the real reasons why we're drinking. But identifying these is a big part of being fully aware of the problem. So have a think about yours.

Do you need a drink to signal the switch from being 'on' to relaxing? (Into this category falls post-work drinks or opening a bottle straight after putting the kids to bed.)

Do you feel that your social life depends on booze, and everything from gossip to problems, to encouragement, is shared over a bottle with friends?

Do you simply enjoy the taste of a nice red wine with your dinner?

Perhaps you're a habitual drinker who has become so used to opening a bottle of wine at home every evening that it would feel extremely weird not to.

Perhaps you're using alcohol to manage your emotions, drinking to numb feelings of stress, anxiety, anger, boredom or loneliness.

Whatever the reasons – and it could be a combination of several – notice them without judgement. Easier said than done, right? The key to being less judgemental with yourself comes from remembering that your brain has been programmed over a lifetime to associate drinking with fun, celebration and stress relief. It's perfectly natural that you want to reach for a bottle of wine after a bad day at work, but this process is all about spotting the feeling, and understanding it, before we can tackle it head on. As we get into how to live more mindfully, this will become easier.

Georgia Foster, the hypnotist I mentioned before, specialises in over-drinking and has identified different personality types that can help you see more clearly the reasons why you drink, two of which sound like so many of my friends it's as if she's stalked my WhatsApp groups.

The first is The Perfectionist; this person struggles with moderation because of an all-or-nothing attitude. 'They're high-achievers, they're very interested in how they look, they probably eat healthily and exercise all week,' explains Foster, 'and they're able to abstain from Monday to Thursday, but then it's their justification for binge-drinking at the weekend. So when they do drink, because they're so diligent in other areas of their life, their inner critic will kick in. That negative voice says: "You're going to drink too much tonight. What's your problem? Everybody else is moderate but you." It becomes a self-fulfilling prophecy because, once they start to worry that they have a problem, there's more anxiety, which leads to more drinking. And because there are high levels of anxiety, they drink really quickly. They'll have had two glasses of wine when everyone else is still on their first.'

The second personality type that Foster talks me through is The Pleaser, and this is the one that is close to the bone for me.

I'm such a hopeless people-pleaser that when a car stops for me at a zebra crossing, I do a little jog across the road so I don't hold them up too much. If a friend says something like, 'I don't want to drink on my own' or 'Go on, it's my birthday,' I don't stand a chance. Although The Pleaser never appears to lose control, she actually drinks more than The Perfectionist, who is quite capable of going out to drinks on a Tuesday night and sticking with San Pellegrino because she's got an early start in the morning. 'But The Pleaser will be coerced,' says Foster, 'because they don't want to feel that they're offending or rejecting. The Pleaser doesn't really have any alcohol-free days. They don't want to stop the party.'

Another category that comes through in Foster's work is The Inner Child, which manifests in most of us to a greater or lesser extent. This is the personality type that pays no attention to what they *should* be doing, and is very selective about the word 'no'. Once alcohol has numbed your inhibitions, your Inner Child may well come out in the form of anger or tears, or even just ill-intended office gossip. This part of your personality needs to be nurtured and made to feel safe, because the negative side of your Inner Child comes from a place of fear. So working out the emotional issues behind a person's alcohol intake is key. As Foster says: 'It's a thinking problem, not a drinking problem.'

You might not fall neatly into one of these trigger categories, but I bet you loosely associate with one more than the other. And at the root of all of these personality types is anxiety. 'In America, you've got a pharmacy on every corner,' says Foster, referring to the fact that one in six Americans is on medication for anxiety or depression,[9] 'but in the UK, you've got a pub on every corner. It's how we manage our vulnerabilities and negativity, whether that's anything from social anxiety to financial pressures.'

You thought buying this book would help you drink less alcohol, and it will, but to get there we need to deal with the underlying anxiety which, frankly, is the main issue here. Then we can go about changing your life.

ANXIETY

One in four people in the UK will experience a mental health problem each year,[10] anxiety and depression being the most common. But the word 'anxiety' covers a ridiculously broad range of human emotions. It's that gnawing feeling in the back of your head when you know there's something you forgot to do at work today. It's the jitters you get before an exam, or a date, or a job interview. It's also the flooding, debilitating dread of a panic attack. Wherever you are on this spectrum, no two cases are ever the same, and there is no one-size-fits-all answer.

If you're anything like me, a glass of wine has been your anxiety quick-fix for as long as you can remember. This is because

9 The Medical Expenditure Panel Survey, 2013
10 The NHS Information Centre for Health and Social Care, 2017

alcohol slows down your brain, which feels relaxing because it stalls your anxious thoughts. But, long term, regular drinking interferes with neurotransmitters and lowers the level of serotonin in our brains, making the stress problem worse.

Anxiety and depression are more common in heavy drinkers, and heavy drinking is more common in those with anxiety and depression. It's a vicious circle, and one that is so common it now has a name: 'hangxiety'.

'Anxiety is absolutely a key cause in drinking too much,' says Lauren Booker, a consultant, trainer and coach for Alcohol Concern. 'It's something that really needs to be acknowledged. Because we fear anxiety so much, but it's OK to feel a bit anxious. Live through it. You'll realise it's not so bad. I managed. I coped. And I did it without the fear of saying or doing something embarrassing because of drinking too much. If you can face those anxieties and sit with them, they lose their power. Anxiety is part of life. It's normal. We need to demystify it, and then it won't have the power to make you paralysed with fear.'

But for some people anxiety is a huge issue, and resisting the urge to numb those feelings with alcohol is far easier said than done.

'It is very easy to say that someone should do x, y and z to address their patterns of over-drinking, but the mind of an anxious person is a tangle of shoulds and associated coping mechanisms,' says Eleanor Morgan, author of *Anxiety For Beginners*. 'Patterns can be tricky to break. The key is acceptance and self-compassion.

It is important that the person who over-drinks is helped

a compassionate voice towards their experiences. It is

fault for wanting to numb distressing feelings. There is n

in wanting to not feel terrible, but we owe it to ourselves to try to

manage our feelings in a way that doesn't make us feel worse in

the long run.'

So although for some people this is a much bigger moun-tain to climb, the answer is still in accepting anxiety as a part of life.

'Over time, it is very possible to learn to manage anxiety,' ex-plains Morgan. 'The key is learning – which may take time – to accept your propensity for it and that, aside from acute episodes, to be alive is to experience undulations in mood and mindset all the time. It's how we develop resilience for the low or anxious moments that makes a difference.'

Sitting through uncomfortable feelings is a big part of this process. Urges and cravings make you feel as though they must be satisfied immediately, so learning to sit with the discomfort of wanting a drink but not giving in to that urge is a powerful skill. It's also important to look after yourself in other ways. Ways that might not initially seem related to your anxiety. If you have the flu or break a leg, you understand that your body needs time to heal, and things like nourishing food and enough sleep will help the process. It's the same for your mind – it takes time and self-care to deal with difficult mental states.

Work-related stress is one of the biggest causes of anxiety.

Alcohol is the socially acceptable drug to use as a coping mechanism,' says Laura Willoughby of Club Soda. 'I was always a big drinker but my drinking escalated when I was in a job where I didn't feel that I was valued. I took the only tool I had and abused it totally.'

It's a pattern that many people will recognise. Work stress has always been a huge issue in terms of reasons why people drink too much, but the world is changing faster than our brains can adapt. And, now that we're all so connected 24/7, we never really switch off from work. The best way to deal with it is to sit down and think hard about what it is that's actually making you stressed.

Is there something you forgot to do today? Something you did wrong? Something you just thought of that you need to deal with tomorrow? Whatever it is, decide what you need to do about it, and write it down. The act of writing it down moves the problem from your brain to the page. And focusing on the practicalities of whatever it is you're worried about will help prevent you opening a bottle of wine to try to forget about it.

Another big way in which anxiety leads us to drink is social situations. Social anxiety inflicts us all at one point or another, although for some it can be significantly more severe.

'For an anxious person, there is often a great fight between however your symptoms manifest and the need to feel connected and "normal", so they drink in order to facilitate sociability,' says Eleanor Morgan. 'The downside is that alcohol can be a potent depressive – particularly in those who have a predisposition to depression and anxiety. You feel compelled to not miss out on life because that would mean "giving in" to the anxiety, so you drink anyway, even though you know it will make you feel terrible later on. This may be particularly true for people who find it difficult to accept that their mental health can waver in this way,' she continues. 'They feel they "need" alcohol to loosen up or feel a buzz that knocks the edges off their nerves.'

Learning to do without that crutch can feel overwhelming, so I contacted someone who knows a thing or two about the problems of dealing with social situations while sober.

British writer Ruby Warrington has a background in fashion journalism, which meant a booze-fuelled party-girl lifestyle. After moving to New York, she overhauled her life, cutting out alcohol almost entirely.

'In the long term, overcoming social anxiety could mean digging deep into the factors eating away at your self-confidence,' she tells me. 'This is the real root of social anxiety, and it can be a lifetime's work. It's essentially about identifying who you really are, and getting comfortable living as this authentic self, despite societal pressures to conform.'

But first, explains Warrington, we must 'unlearn' a lifetime of conditioning that you need to drink alcohol to have fun. 'Alcohol is a highly addictive substance that is marketed aggressively at us with megabucks ad campaigns, the same way cigarettes used to be. It would be very hard for it not to have become ingrained in our culture,' she says. 'Especially as the key "problems" it appears to solve for us – lack of confidence, social anxiety, general unhappiness, lack of joy, stress – are commonplace in a society that offers very narrow and rigid ideas about what it means to be successful, social, or cool.'

We've all heard of Dutch courage, but using alcohol to numb your inhibitions does not make you more confident. All it does is prevent you learning real confidence, which comes with getting through stressful situations while sober. When we get to your clean break, I'll take you through how to learn and practise sober socialising. Once you've done it, you'll feel bulletproof.

MODERATION VS ABSTINENCE

When it comes to drinking, many people are able to quit completely for a certain period – if they're pregnant or doing Dry January, for example. But long-term moderation is more difficult, for two reasons. First of all, abstinence provides a clear line with no possibility of it becoming blurred. This prevents indecision around, shall I drink today? What shall I drink? How much shall I drink? Moderation involves many decisions, all of which provide an opportunity to slip up. The second reason is that, once you have had one or two drinks, your iron will dissolves. Alcohol hits the pleasure centre of your brain, which makes the 'off-switch' in your mind a bit tricky to reach. This is why your alcohol-free days will actually be easier to get through than the days when you allow yourself to drink.

Gretchen Rubin tells me that people broadly fall into two categories: abstainers and moderators. Moderators hate the idea of depriving themselves of something (cake, prosecco, a guilty browse of celebrity gossip), so will have a little bit of whatever it is, but never overdo it. Abstainers, meanwhile, struggle to only have a little of something:

'Oh my, that cake was good, is there any more?'

'Shall we open another bottle?'

'I only wanted to see Nicole Kidman's Oscars dress but have fallen down a Sidebar of Shame spiral and now I'm looking at a Towie star on the beach!'

By this rationale, I'm an abstainer: I find it much easier to have no chocolate than a small piece. I'll either politely decline your offer of a Malteser, or accept one and then immediately have to go out and buy a bag of my own. (Who are those people who keep a bar of chocolate in their desk drawer and have one square a day? I find that unfathomable!) But when it comes to alcohol, I didn't want to abstain. I wanted to learn how to be moderate. I asked Rubin if she thinks that's even possible: can an abstainer learn to be a moderater?

'If you're an abstainer it's much easier to abstain completely, so a better way to think about it is "planned exceptions",' she explains. 'So you're going to generally abstain, because trying to have half a glass of wine every night wouldn't work for you. But you can tell yourself, "I'm not saying I'm never going to drink again." You can make a planned exception. The important thing is to plan it in advance, so you're in control. You can look forward to it and anticipate it with pleasure. You can experience it and feel good about it and, when you look back on it, you can feel that you kept your word to yourself. If you drink when you didn't intend to, because you made some excuse on the spur of the moment, then you'll feel that you let yourself down and look back on it with regret. You'll feel like you're not in control of yourself, and that's a bad feeling.'

The good news is, Rubin says it will get easier with time. 'People think that if they deny themselves something the cravings will build,' she says. 'In my experience, cravings diminish the longer you go without it.'

This idea makes sense because, by its very nature, drinking makes you want to drink. Therefore, even those who are able to be moderate in other parts of their lives might struggle with moderate drinking. David Crane, of University College London's Department of Behavioural Science and Health, explains it like this: 'Once people have consumed one drink, that can activate programmed responses to alcohol, and deactivate inhibition. In other words, consuming alcohol itself can make people want to drink more. We suggest having days off alcohol as a better way of cutting down.'

If the thought of alcohol-free days fills you with dread, you need an incentive.

THE PROBLEM IN A NUTSHELL

- Moderation is harder than abstinence because it requires constant awareness.
- It also provides many opportunities to backslide, since drinking disables your off-switch.
- Alcohol-free days will become very important once we get on to how to moderate your drinking.
- Being aware of the huge role of anxiety in over-drinking will help identify triggers and pitfalls.
- Changing your drinking identity is going to require a reinvention.
- Drinking alcohol is socially ingrained in everything from celebration to stress relief, and it's even worse if you're a woman. So remember: it's *not* your fault.

NOTES

....
....
....
....
....
....
....
....
....
....
....
....
....
....
....
....
....
....
....
....
....
....
....
....
....

2

THE INCENTIVE

Before you read this section, I want to be clear that my aim is absolutely not to be preachy or scaremongering, but simply to inform. Read on with a positive mindset. Yes, hearing about the negative effects of your much-loved glass of wine might sound depressing, but you are on the cusp of changing your life in a really positive way.

Many people are unaware of the full extent of the damage that alcohol can cause. Or perhaps they're deliberately ignoring this inconvenient truth – I know I used to. Back in 2010, a British study published in *The Lancet*[11] rated legal and illegal drugs in order of which cause the most harm. They analysed everything from damage to health and likelihood of developing a dependency to it, to things like the economic cost. Which one do you think came out on top? Yep, alcohol. It was deemed more harmful than crack, meth, tobacco, cocaine and heroin.

11 By the Independent Scientific Committee on Drugs

It can happen that warning someone about the dangers of alcohol only makes them want to drink. It's a form of rebellion, and I totally get it. Particularly when your unconscious mind still believes that you need alcohol for fun, so part of you still thinks cutting back is about deprivation. Knowing the dangers of alcohol, yet still craving it, can be extremely uncomfortable emotionally because it causes two parts of your mind to be at war with one another. And the way in which our feelings influence our thoughts and behaviour is so subtle and pervasive that you wouldn't normally even know it was happening. That's why it's important to know the facts before we go any further. The more you know about the negative effects of alcohol, the easier it becomes to control your drinking, rather than letting it control you.

Annie Grace is the author of *This Naked Mind: Control Alcohol: Find Freedom, Discover Happiness & Change Your Life*, a comprehensive study of the way that our unconscious beliefs about alcohol are largely responsible for our over-drinking. 'Liminal Thinking is one of the ways I use to uncover my own unconscious desires,' she says. 'The process is quite simple, yet profound. You look at what you believe, simply stating that belief – for example, "alcohol relaxes me". Then you question what experiences you have had and what assumptions you have made to form this belief. This is important as you need to understand where you formed this idea.'

So if your belief is that alcohol enhances your life, you can look at the endless media messages correlating drinking with celebration, socialising and the end of loneliness. The next step is to find out if there is any solid evidence to support your belief. 'I did this by starting to research if alcohol is relaxing,' explains Grace. 'Consciously examining external evidence is pivotal to changing the unconscious.'

This is where The Incentive comes in, and it's a fundamental part of the process because you need solid reasons behind your desire to change. Most people who have a serious drinking problem tend to have a 'rock bottom' moment before they get help. If, like me, you want to drink less but have never actually woken up in a gutter, it can be easy to slide back into your old habits because drinking never seemed to affect your life in such a dramatic way. Of course, you can think of ways in which to reward yourself for not drinking, which I'll come to later, but ultimately you have to *want* to drink less. And after this section, I guarantee you will. Some of the points made here will strike a chord with you more than others, and while it might be a tough read, I promise you it's worth it.

YOUR SKIN

OK, let's start with one of the most effective ways to make people sit up and pay attention. I'm going to appeal to your vanity. I will happily admit that I'm pretty vain, and it was only when I noticed after a heavy night that alcohol was beginning to impact my skin that I finally started to worry about it. I distinctly remember doing my eyeliner before a work event, having barely recovered from the previous night's drinks, and wondering when my eyelids got so ... droopy.

You might have heard of the phenomenon known as Wine Face. Of course, it can actually be brought on by all types of alcohol, not just wine. Dehydration causes wrinkles, which is why heavy drinkers often have pronounced frown lines, while the high sugar content damages collagen production, making skin saggy (hello jowls!). Add in enlarged pores, droopy eyelids and a reddish, uneven skin tone and you're causing problems that no expensive facialist can solve.

But your skin is an amazing organ, and its regenerative powers make Doctor Who look lazy. Drinking lots of water, and having alcohol-free days to give your skin a break, will rehydrate your face and bring back that glow. I noticed a difference in my skin within weeks, and smugly enjoyed people telling me I looked remarkably fresh-faced for someone with two young children.

YOUR BRAIN

The reason why you feel good after one or two drinks is because alcohol suppresses activity in the prefrontal cortex; the part of your brain that controls inhibition. In a nutshell, that means you give less of a shit about things that might otherwise have concerned you. However, the prefrontal cortex also controls things like problem solving, decision making and social behaviour, which is why you might wake up with a head full of regrets the next day.

Dopamine is the neurotransmitter that is responsible for cravings. When you have an alcoholic drink (or any addictive substance – drugs work in the same way), the dopamine that is released makes you feel relaxed. But it's an artificial stimulation of your 'reward centre' rather than an authentic burst of joy – such as a laugh with a good friend or a hug with someone you love. And, unfortunately, heavy drinking has been shown to deplete dopamine levels to the extent that the drinker needs more and more alcohol to get the same buzz,[12] and may also struggle to find joy in other parts of their lives. Dopamine depletion is associated with tiredness, lack of concentration, forgetfulness, anxiety, insomnia, low motivation and full-on depression.

Booze is a depressant, which means it makes your brain processes slow down, leading to both short- and long-term memory loss. Glutamate and GABA are the key neurotransmitters here. To make a memory stick, the brain needs to increase glutamate and decrease GABA, but alcohol has the opposite effect on both these neurotransmitters. It inhibits glutamate, which is why your reactions are slower and your speech is slurred, while boosting

12 A 2016 study published in *Proceedings of the National Academy of Sciences*

GABA, which has a sedative effect. In doing so, alcohol is literally stealing your memories. That regret you feel when you wake up? Sometimes you might not even remember exactly why you have it. That's 'beer fear', and it's a particularly icky feeling. These days, I love waking up after a night out with a clear recollection of the evening and zero fear that I might have accidentally offended someone with a drunken remark. If only the 25-year-old me had known that was even possible.

Anything we do regularly creates a neurological pathway in our brains. This is how habits are formed. It can be simple, obvious patterns, such as opening a bottle of wine at home every night. But it can also mean the way in which the heavy drinking we did at university (while thinking, 'this is just what students do, I'll get my shit together when I graduate') quickly becomes familiar so that our brains are inclined to fall back on that behaviour throughout our adult lives. How often have you said 'yes' to a glass of wine, simply because it was expected, rather than thinking about whether it's what you actually want? I've done that more times than I can count.

But new neurological pathways can always be forged. We can establish new healthy habits by repeating them often enough to break them into our brains. It takes effort and commitment initially, but once something has become a habit, it is like second nature. I'll come to the details later on, but for now, just know that your brain is not against you. In fact, it can be your greatest ally in establishing more alcohol-free days and more self-control when you do drink. This in turn will mean more energy, less anxiety, improved moods, better concentration and fewer regrets.

YOUR FINANCES

It's only in the last few decades that is has become normal to have alcoholic drinks at home, and standard to open a bottle of wine with dinner. Even just 40 years ago, wine was for special occasions, not to accompany a Tuesday night bowl of pasta and pesto. Supermarkets regularly have deals on that make you think you're saving money, but, as I always try to tell myself when browsing through the Whistles sale, it's not a bargain if you don't need it.

Drinking at home is expensive enough, but if you regularly buy drinks in a bar, even only once or twice a week, you could be drinking away anywhere in the region of £1,500–3,000 a year – even more if you live in a city like London, where one gin and tonic can easily cost a tenner.

When I was pregnant and would go out for a booze-free dinner, I was always shocked at how cheap the bill was. Not drinking means you can enjoy an amazing meal in an incredible restaurant for a comparatively reasonable price.

Try keeping a diary of your expenditure and separate out the money that you spend on alcohol. You'll find it's the most expensive part of any meal, the most expensive bit of your Ocado order. Arguably more important than the financial cost, is time. A 2017 study[13] found that spending money on things to buy you time (such as taking a taxi or getting a cleaner) is the quickest route to happiness. Alcohol robs you of time. It makes you forget entire evenings, it makes mornings a write-off. So it's easy to see how saving time *and* money simply by drinking less will vastly improve your quality of life.

SEX

You know by now that alcohol suppresses your inhibitions, which can make you feel frisky, so that initially sounds like good news for your sex life (assuming you're not finding yourself in inappropriate or dangerous sexual situations). But any more than very moderate drinking can cause serious problems. It is widely known that alcohol is the main cause of sexual dysfunction in men, including low sexual desire, erectile dysfunction and, oddly, both premature and delayed ejaculation. Fewer people know that, in women, it decreases sexual desire and deadens the senses, leading to difficulty in reaching orgasm and decreased intensity of orgasm. Also, the dehydrating effects of alcohol can mean less, er, natural lubrication. So take a moment to think about how many times you have

13 Buying Time Promotes Happiness, 2017, *Proceedings of the National Academy of Sciences*

actually had sex sober (and the morning after a boozy night doesn't count). If you've been missing out on sober sex, now's the time to try it because, while the disinhibiting effect of a glass of wine or two might make you feel libidinous, the actual sex is significantly better with no alcohol in your system. And, of course, you are far less likely to regret a sober sexual encounter than you are one where alcohol was clouding your judgement.

SOCIABILITY

This is an area where many people believe that alcohol is not just harmless but sometimes necessary. People believe their friends will feel judged or offended in some way if they don't drink. They also believe that the effect of alcohol on their inhibitions makes them more fun on a night out.

But let's deconstruct those beliefs.

Inhibitions are nothing to be afraid of. They exist for a reason. It's your inhibitions that stop you ripping off all your clothes on the dance floor, or telling your boss they've got control issues, or taking a shortcut down that spooky dark alleyway. Inhibitions and anxiety are closely related and it's just as important to acknowledge your inhibitions as it is your anxiety, rather than numbing these feelings with alcohol. You're not funnier, or more confident, when drunk, you're simply less aware of your behaviour, which means you're more likely to say something stupid or to offend.

In many situations, you probably feel more confident after a couple of drinks, but, paradoxically, drinking actually makes you *less* confident in the long term, and eventually it makes you feel like withdrawing from socialising as much as possible. This is because confidence is something that comes with experience, and if you rarely experience social situations while sober your confidence doesn't get a chance to grow. Sober socialising will bring you the real, authentic confidence that only comes with having the courage to break through the fear of entering social situations without that crutch.

Drinking less alcohol makes you a more empathetic listener, a more articulate anecdotalist and more capable of remembering what happened the next day. As a result, your relationships will become more authentic and fulfilling. Plus, nobody likes hanging out with the friend they have to bundle into a taxi because they can barely stand at the end of the night.

If you genuinely feel that you can't have fun in a social situation without alcohol, take a good look at where you are, who you're with and whether there is any joy to be found there. Believe me, if you struggle to find joy in a social situation, it is not the lack of alcohol to blame.

The friends that needed me to drink with them, in order to make themselves feel better, fell away from my social life quite quickly after I started drinking less. But the friends worth keeping were happy to have a sober evening with me, or enjoy their drinks without caring whether I was drinking or not. Cultivate friendships where you can go out for dinner or to the cinema and just have one drink, if any, because it simply doesn't matter. Those friends are the keepers.

WORK

Annie Grace found her drinking escalated when she was in a job with a big boozy culture. 'I actually thought drinking was key to my career,' she explains, 'but I became more of a gossip after a few drinks and often wondered what I had said the following morning, which caused a huge amount of stress.' Not only that, but Grace found she was drinking to deal with work stress in ways that were less than helpful. 'If I was worried about a large presentation or report, I would have a few drinks – instead of preparing the report,' she admits. 'It made me feel less stressed in the moment but only actually doing the work both relieved my stress and made it so that I was advancing my career.' These days, she doesn't drink at all. 'I was very afraid of the work-related backlash after I stopped drinking, but most of it was in my mind,' she says. 'People were supportive and accepting. I ended up doing better in my career after giving up alcohol than before.'

Her experience makes sense. If you have ever sat at your desk staring blankly at your computer screen, praying the coffee will kick in soon so you can gather your thoughts enough to reply to an email, then you know how one too many can affect your performance at work. I know I'm not alone in this. In fact, one in ten British people go to work with a hangover at least twice a week.[14]

'Coming down' is phrase normally reserved for drug use, but alcohol *is* a drug, and coming down the morning after a night of heavy drinking causes anxiety and paranoia. There are hardly any clinical studies in this area, due to the ethical implications of getting people drunk to study the damage to their brain, so the evidence is either anecdotal or from studies where the drinking is 'naturalistic' – i.e. the subjects just drink what they normally would. This, of course, means the results are less precise, but various studies have shown the mental after-effects include regret, low mood and anxiety.[15] (Although it doesn't take a scientist to tell that to anyone who's had a hangover.)

This is why 'hair of the dog' is so tempting, since that dopamine hit will instantly make you feel better. That's generally difficult to do in the workplace, though, unless your office is like *Mad Men*. Besides your mood, other symptoms of a hangover, such as fatigue, anxiety and lack of concentration, pale in comparison to the long-term effects of heavy drinking. Bad judgement and

14 Drinkaware
15 A review of the next day effects of alcohol on subjective mood ratings, 2010, University of Ulster

poor problem-solving skills, along with indecisiveness, lack of confidence and paranoia, will make colleagues less inclined to add you to that meeting invitation.

If you like your job, surely you want to give it your all and be the sharpest, most motivated, confident version of yourself in the office? And if you don't, you need energy, decisiveness and drive to either make it work for you or find something else. Just getting through the day in a hung-over haze, and looking forward to your glass of wine at the end of it, is really not doing you any favours.

SLEEP

Many people believe that alcohol actually helps them sleep. 'That misconception exists because the immediate sensation you get when drinking alcohol is that you feel drowsy and sleepy,' says Dr John Larsen, Director of Evidence and Impact at the charity Drinkaware. 'Alcohol is a depressant drug, and that feeling of not-so-alertness can make you fall asleep more quickly.'

Also, alcohol numbs your mind, which enables you to – however briefly – forget about your worries. This is another reason why it's easier to drop off after a couple of drinks: alcohol presses pause on that whirring carousel of thoughts and anxieties.

'However,' Dr Larsen continues, 'if you have alcohol in your system the quality of your sleep is not good. You don't get the deep, restorative sleep, so when you wake up, you don't feel refreshed. You haven't been through the deep-sleep phases. Even if you don't have a hangover, your sleep will have been affected.'

So drinking interferes with your sleep cycles, which explains why you pass out easily at 11.30 p.m., then are wide awake, with all your anxieties back tenfold, at 3.30 a.m.. Then 7.30 a.m. comes around and it feels like the world's biggest effort to drag yourself into the shower.

Logically, I knew that alcohol didn't help my sleep but, after a stressful day at work, I found it too easy to reach for a glass of wine to quieten my mind and help me drop off – conveniently forgetting about the wide-awake 3 a.m. panic.

Unfortunately, if your perception is that you will sleep better after a few drinks, even though that is not the case, it easily becomes a bad habit. Increasingly you will feel incredibly tired at the end of the day and, desperate for sleep, you drink again. And, of course, lacking a proper night's sleep leads not only to fatigue throughout the day but also to bad skin, bad moods and bad choices.

Drinking less alcohol will transform your sleep, delivering a proper, healing rest for your mind and body, making you feel like a new person in the morning.

YOUR BODY

Alcoholic drinks account for 11 per cent of the UK population's daily intake of added sugar. A 250ml glass of wine contains 228 calories, roughly equivalent to a bar of chocolate or an ice-cream. Imagine how gross you'd feel (and look) if you regularly ate three or four ice-creams in one evening. Drinking five pints of lager a week adds up to 44,200 calories over a year, equivalent to eating 221 doughnuts. Feeling queasy yet?

You probably already knew that drinking makes you fat, but it's less likely that you were fully aware of the effects on your gut. Many people suffer from a range of issues that are often loosely diagnosed as Irritable Bowel Syndrome (IBS): abdominal pain, bloating, wind and constipation or diarrhoea. Sexy, right? Alcohol is a gastrointestinal irritant that contributes to a whole litany of digestion issues, from inflammation and bloating to stomach cramps and anything that comes under the IBS umbrella.

Avoiding weight gain and bloating might almost be enough of an incentive, depending on your own particular body issues. Of course, moderating heavy drinking will help protect you from many more serious conditions, such as high blood pressure, liver disease and cardiovascular problems. Drinking less will also make you less likely to pick up infections, since over-drinking weakens your immune system.

Then there's cancer. This is the part that makes for particularly bleak reading. The World Health Organization's International Agency for Research on Cancer has classified alcohol as a Group 1 carcinogen. As you might imagine, that is not the best kind of carcinogen.

This is something that we *all* have to take seriously, since half of us are likely to be diagnosed with cancer at some point in our lifetime.[16]

Every year, alcohol causes around 12,800 cases of cancer in the UK, which is about 4 per cent of all cancers. Surprisingly, liver cancer is far from the most common. The numbers are biggest for cancers of the mouth and throat, as well as bowel and breast cancer (around 3,200 cases of breast cancer in the UK are linked to alcohol use every year).[17] Women who consume two to five drinks a day are 40 per cent more likely to get breast cancer than non-drinkers. In fact, just one drink a day can raise a woman's cancer risk by about 7 per cent,[18] which is part of the reason why alcohol-free days are so important in your new mindful drinking life.

One 2017 study[19] went so far as to accuse the alcohol industry of 'denial, distortion, distraction' tactics in an effort to cover up the link to cancer, likening it to the decades-long cancer-cover-up

16 Cancer Research UK
17 Cancer Research UK
18 British Journal of Cancer
19 By the London School of Hygiene and Tropical Medicine

behaviour of the tobacco industry. The study even went on to say that the close link to breast cancer in particular has been glossed over – despite over 100 studies between 2007 and 2017 proving it – since women are such big consumers of alcohol.

The good news (and we need some here) is that it appears to be a sliding scale, meaning that any reduction in alcohol intake will reduce your risk of getting cancer.

BUT THERE ARE SOME HEALTH BENEFITS OF DRINKING, RIGHT?

You've probably seen news articles shared on Facebook with headlines like 'Having A Drink May Help You Live Longer'[20] or 'The Unexpected Health Benefits Of Red Wine.'[21] Stories like this are shared liberally, with lots of likes and wine glass emojis. Some good news at last in the bleak cycle of war and terrorism on the internet! No wonder people cling to them like a life raft. I know I've certainly clicked 'like' on plenty of them in the past.

But for every story saying red wine is good for your heart, there is another refuting it. There was recently a big study jointly conducted by researchers from Oxford University and UCL,

20 *Time*, 2017
21 *Telegraph*, 2017

concluding that even moderate drinking can damage the brain.[22] And then there was the report by medical group United European Gastroenterology that put British people among the most at-risk in Europe for alcohol-related cancer.[23] Didn't see either of those shared on social media, did you? Psychologists call this 'confirmation bias'. It's our tendency to click and share stories that support what we believe, or want to believe. Another issue, of course, is that lots of the positive studies are funded by the alcohol industry. Hmm . . . dubious.

'There is lots of different research coming out all the time and it can be really confusing for the public,' acknowledges Dr Larsen of Drinkaware. 'And the media is quite happy to jump on things, so they don't help with that because they exaggerate it. When you look at the bigger picture, as was recently done in a big review, there are not any overall health benefits of drinking.'

The truth is, in terms of the health-boosting antioxidants that people often say are in red wine, you're really better off eating a bunch of red grapes or a handful of blueberries. But then you already knew that, didn't you?

So if alcohol is so bad for us, why is this book about moderation, rather than abstinence? Shouldn't I be encouraging people to give up rather than cut down? The way I see it is this: I know that sugar is bad for me, and cake offers no health benefits whatsoever, but if it's your birthday and you present me with a slice of

22 Published in the *British Medical Journal*, 2017
23 *The Guardian*, 2017

Konditor & Cook's Lemon Chiffon Cake, damn right I'm eating it. The pleasure I get from eating that slice of cake, for me, negates the adverse health effects. I just make sure that I enjoy every bite, and I don't eat cake every day. This is how it ought to be with alcohol, too. I know that, in a perfect world, I wouldn't drink at all. But we don't live in a perfect world, and I'm a big fan of the power of 'good enough'.

If, after reading this book, you find that you want to cut out alcohol entirely and you believe that you can, great – go ahead. But I didn't want to lose alcohol from my life altogether. I just wanted to have a healthier relationship with it. And keeping these incentives in mind helps me make a better, more informed, more mindful decision about every single drink that passes my lips.

THE CUT-OUT-AND-KEEP INCENTIVE LIST

By moderating my drinking I will have:

- Clearer, firmer, glowing skin
- Increased energy
- Sharpened concentration
- Fewer regrets
- Improved memory
- Extra disposable income
- Better sex
- Less anxiety
- Improved moods
- Deeper, more restorative sleep
- Greater motivation and productivity at work
- Weight loss
- More authentic, fulfilling relationships
- Improved digestion
- Stronger immune system
- Smaller risk of developing cancer.

NOTES

3

PREPARATION

Now you understand the problem, and you have the incentive to do something about it, we're going to lay the groundwork for your new relationship with alcohol. Planning and preparation are key to this process, but just as important is awareness. The ability to acknowledge the emotional reasons behind your desire to drink alcohol, and to be capable of drinking it consciously, knowing when to stop, is something that comes with the practice of mindfulness.

Dr Sunjeev Kamboj, Deputy Director of the Clinical Psychopharmacology Unit at UCL, recently oversaw a study that analysed whether mindfulness could help reduce alcohol intake in heavy drinkers. 'There's a growing evidence base showing that mindfulness is effective in preventing relapse in addicts, but we were curious to know whether giving participants really brief instructions on how to do mindfulness would have any beneficial effects on problematic drinking,' he tells me. 'By doing a carefully controlled laboratory study, we were able to look at the specific effects of mindfulness, and we found that participants reduced their drinking by about the equivalent of a bottle of wine in the week after being given the instructions.'

Interestingly, the subjects of the study weren't actually trying to reduce their consumption; they were simply chosen because they drank more than the recommended guidelines. But the reduction in alcohol intake happened anyway – and this was with nothing but the regular use of an 11-minute guided meditation recording.

'It's encouraging that such a brief set of instructions can have a measurable effect on consumption,' says Kamboj, although he is keen to add that it's unlikely to be a stand-alone treatment for those with more severe alcohol use disorder, who might need to be supported by suitable medical or psychological treatments. Having said that, 'brief mindfulness instructions can shift people's drinking habits, and might help to kick-start a process of change'. It certainly helped me, simply by increasing my awareness around alcohol. And there are many little ways in which mindfulness has now become a big part of my life.

But first, let's clear up any confusion about the difference between 'mindfulness' and 'meditation'. Meditation is generally considered to mean the formal practice of sitting in quiet contemplation. Whereas mindfulness, while also requiring awareness and presence, is often thought of as something that it's possible to apply to specific areas of your life – for example, mindful eating, mindful parenting, mindful breathing and, of course, mindful drinking.

The reason why people who meditate are often heard extolling the ways in which the practice has made them calmer, happier and more successful is because it declutters a person's mind and helps them see things more clearly. When you can see a glass of wine for what it is – i.e. not a magic fun potion that forges friendships and improves your mood, but a sugary, acidic drink that is toxic if you have too much – it helps you decide more easily if you want one.

'There is a huge body of scientific evidence that supports the idea that mindfulness strengthens the pre-frontal cortex,' says Annie Grace, author of *This Naked Mind*. 'This is the exact part of your brain that is damaged by alcohol and that allows us to make better decisions. For that reason alone I believe it is an important tool in the exploration of one's relationship with alcohol. There are numerous other benefits – such as reduced stress and anxiety – which are often the reasons we drink more than we intend in the first place.'

Mindfulness techniques can make you keenly aware of habitual patterns of behaviour. Not only that, but a sense of presence opens the door to controlling your cravings. This is because you can't control what you don't acknowledge, and mindfulness is all about being aware of your thoughts and feelings and acknowledging them, without judgement. It helps you react to things in a more positive way. Through mindfulness, something internal becomes external, because you can see your reactions very clearly. So, in the past, I would have poured and knocked back a glass of wine after a stressful day, without giving it a moment's thought. Mindfulness helps me see the stress for what it is, and make a better decision about how to deal with it.

Rohan Gunatillake is the creator of bestselling meditation app buddhify, and the author of *Modern Mindfulness.* He tells me how, while writing, he kept being distracted by his phone. So he decided to treat the process of distraction mindfully, and get to the root of what was causing it. The answer was not his phone – in the same way that what causes over-drinking is not the drink itself.

'I started catching it earlier and earlier in the process,' he explains. 'And eventually I was able to notice what my mind state was at the moment before the distraction happened. I was always feeling a bit lonely or bored or restless, or frustrated with what I was doing. That was the primary problem, and I was checking my email to make myself feel better.'

Whether it's checking Instagram or having a drink, we do it to temporarily numb an anxious feeling. Mindfulness helps you interrupt your unconscious brain's belief that drinking will help your anxiety with your rational brain's understanding that, long term, it really won't.

Right now you're probably thinking that this is another thing you have to learn, another thing to think about, another thing to clog up your life, which is far too full of *things* already. If that's how you feel, I fully understand, because I was there too.

Seduced by the many benefits of meditation, I tried to get into it several times over the years. I'd listen to Oprah Winfrey and Deepak Chopra's guided meditations every now and then but, being a busy (and generally hung-over) young journalist, I usually listened while walking from the tube to the office and didn't find that mindfulness helped much with my pavement rage against slow-walking tourists. Later, I was delighted to discover the Headspace app: here was a way of doing meditation that was modern, relevant and stylishly designed. I downloaded and deleted the app from my phone several times, veering between wanting to make meditation a regular practice, then feeling that it's just another thing to remember to do, another app clogging up the memory on my phone.

I know that lots of people feel that way. Either they don't believe they have the time or the patience to sit around and meditate, which was my issue, or they just think it's all a bunch of hippy nonsense. The good news is, there are plenty of ways to be mindful without doing formal seated meditation. It turns out there is such a thing as meditation for people who don't have time to meditate. And this is where Rohan Gunatillake's app, buddhify, comes in. This app is all about incorporating mindfulness into your everyday life. Yes, even *your* everyday life, with that full-on job, hectic social life, creative side-hustle and exhausting family commitments. Not to mention the yoga class you never make it to, the cooking you never get around to, and the friends you don't have time to see. buddhify is designed for people who don't have time. There are short guided meditations for when you're walking in a city, waiting in a queue or having a quick work break, and specific ones for being on a plane, or for when you can't sleep.

'I want to free people from the idea that meditation has to be done in a formal way,' says Gunatillake, whose 'mobile meditation' method is the wrecking ball to demolish that widely held misconception that you have to sit on the floor and close your eyes. I tell Gunatillake that I have struggled in the past because meditation always felt like another thing on my endless to-do list. 'That is the worst,' he sighs. 'It shouldn't feel like a job, or like you're fixing yourself. It should be fun, because you only sustainably learn when you're having fun.'

One of the buddhify techniques for walking through a city is called 'shoot love', in which you randomly fire positive thoughts at strangers (only think them, obviously, don't say them out loud like some kind of weirdo). Try it, and see how much of a better mood it puts you in.

'The number one problem that people have with meditation is that they feel they're not doing it right,' says Gunatillake. 'That's why I like to take the pressure off by doing it alongside other activities in an easy way.' His aim is that ultimately people won't need an app, or guided meditations, because they will have learnt to incorporate mindfulness into everything they do. And doing so will drastically alter your relationship with alcohol, for the better.

Mindfulness is all about being present, and bringing awareness to what you're doing. For this reason, you can do it anywhere, any time. Of course, I'm making this sound easier than it actually is because, at any one moment, there is an army of thoughts, feelings, emails, notifications, people and ideas vying for our attention. The challenge is to focus on one thing at a time. It's a case of priorities, and practice. As with any behaviour, if you repeat it often enough, it will become a habit.

PRACTICE MAKES (YOU REALISE THERE'S NO SUCH THING AS) PERFECT

Think of meditation as exercise for your mind. Some people like the structure and discipline of going to the gym regularly, whereas others hate gyms but they walk everywhere and run up the stairs instead of waiting for the lift. It's a case of finding the method that works for you.

I have found it much easier to incorporate mindful moments into everyday activities, rather than finding the time to do formal seated meditation. But, in an ideal world, you would do a bit of both. So it's worth giving meditation 'proper' a go because if you do find you can fit it in (and drinking less does buy you back some time), it will strengthen your mind and make mindful awareness in other areas of your life come more naturally. If you would like guidance, there are plenty of apps and classes and

YouTube tutorials that will take you through a basic meditation. But you don't actually need them because the core technique is really very simple.

....

TRY THIS:

Sit still, close your eyes and pay close attention to your breathing. Notice how the breath feels as you inhale, and exhale. Is it cold or warm? Do you feel it in your chest or your stomach? Notice your breath without trying to change it in any way.
Now choose a word or phrase that represents calmness – it could be 'peace' or 'love' or 'breathe' – and repeat it in your mind. When your mind wanders, acknowledge that thought (whether it's innocuous, such as 'what's for dinner?' or uncomfortable, such as 'I'm dreading that presentation'), and bring your attention back to your chosen word or mantra.
Do this for as long as feels comfortable.

....

If this is the first time you've done it, the chances are it won't feel comfortable for long. In fact, it will probably feel distinctly uncomfortable to a mind that is accustomed to busyness and distraction. This is meditation, and you might have tried it before and thought, well that's not for me. Many people think they 'can't do' meditation when they first try it, but it's not something that happens instantly. It takes time for the practice to click. That's why it's called a 'practice'. I said it's simple, but I never said it's easy.

Taking time to do this will make you so much more focused and productive in other areas of your life. I know it seems counterintuitive to do nothing to achieve more, but it works. You know the saying 'more haste, less speed?' Well, it's that. You need to slow down to speed up.

One way of forging the habit of meditation practice is to make it a social thing. Meditation does not have to be a solo activity. It never used to be: Buddhist monks always meditated in groups. On both American coasts, drop-in meditation studios like MNDFL in New York and Unplug and The Den in Los Angeles are making a trip to a meditation bar as common as going to the gym. And, like most things that we initially assume are a loony LA fad, the concept is slowly making its way over to the UK. Virgin Active now runs meditation classes alongside the standard spin and yoga (which, incidentally, almost always involves an element of mindfulness), and London's Redemption Bar and Good & Proper Tea shop host meditation and brunch sessions. Signing up for a group class or meditation event has the extra benefit of being a social activity that doesn't involve drinking. Plus, if you paid for something you're way more likely to do it.

One of the main reasons why people struggle to meditate

is the feeling that they're doing it wrong. Once you realise that there is no 'wrong', any activity that helps focus your mind on one thing becomes an opportunity to be mindful. If you're walking, don't listen to music but instead concentrate on your steps. If you're travelling, take a few minutes to concentrate on your breath, rather than idly scrolling through Facebook. Anything creative is perfect for this: art, crafting or knitting, or doing one of those grown-up colouring books. A friend of mine who couldn't get on with meditation is into sound healing. You lie on the floor as noises reverberate around you, grounding you without having to think about your breathing or a mantra.

Find what works for you, and incorporate it into your life on a daily basis. Any kind of mindfulness – whether formal seated meditation or finding mindful moments here and there – will strengthen your mind and your commitment to a healthier relationship with alcohol.

....

TRY THIS

One of the simplest ways to calm your mind is by methodically counting. If you're walking, count your steps. If you're sitting, count your breaths. Doing this gives your mind something to focus on. Don't get frustrated if your mind wanders – that is totally expected – just acknowledge that thought and bring your

*mind back to counting. Simple, right? That is meditating. And it's
your route map to a more mindful life, as well as a more mindful
relationship with alcohol.*

MEDITATION: A WARNING

Some people might warn you against meditation because, since
it's about being really aware of your thoughts, there is a chance it
could bring up some difficult emotions. But you need to see the
problem to be able to deal with it, and as long as you stick to the
less-intense 'pop mindfulness' of apps like Headspace and buddhify, it's unlikely that you'll accidentally dig up any particularly
dark issues that your mind had been repressing.

'Perhaps if you're a deeper practitioner, that may become an
issue,' explains Rohan Gunatillake, 'because it is true that the
further down the rabbit hole you go, the more stuff comes up.
But, actually, the more a person is aware of their pattern of using
alcohol, the more they are able to let go of it.'

Once you can see your anxiety for what it is, you don't even
necessarily have to tackle it head on. The other option is simply
to put your mind somewhere more pleasant, which is a case of
training yourself to use a 'diversion system' (such as focusing on
your breathing) to take you away from difficult emotions.

If, having become aware of your anxiety, you feel it's getting out of control, you can seek medical help. A doctor might well recommend mindfulness, but in the form of an MBSR (mindfulness-based stress reduction) course, which is taught by professionals specialising in clinical anxiety.

The other thing to bear in mind is that, although there are plenty of immediate benefits of meditation, it is not a quick fix. So using it for a specific situation, such as before a night out or at times when you want to reach for the bottle out of stress, doesn't really work if you're not used to it. People say that if mindfulness was a drug, it wouldn't be a painkiller that you take when you need it. It would be something like the contraceptive pill, which only works if you take it regularly.

If you want to change your mind for the long term, you should build in some regular practice, in a way that suits you, and do it whether you're feeling great or miserable, optimistic or anxious. The good news is, continued practice will bring enormous benefits in every part of your life.

Dr Sunjeev Kamboj, who oversaw the study that found mindfulness helped reduce alcohol intake in heavy drinkers, has another caveat for those who feel their drinking has become more of a serious issue. 'Addictions don't occur in a vacuum,' he says. 'Usually people have problems in their relationships or limited social support, or they might never have developed healthy habits, like exercising. People with more severe levels of addiction, especially those with alcohol problems who want to quit, should always get medical advice.'

It's an important note for those who feel the severity of their issue with drinking cannot be solved with moderation. But for those of us who simply want to cut down and have a more thoughtful relationship with alcohol, mindfulness tools can be of enormous benefit. Think of this as a way to anchor you to what's important, giving you a strong sense of self, a solid foundation. So difficult situations, social pressures and tragic events may shake you, but can no longer knock you down. It has changed my life for the better, and it can do the same for you.

....

PERMANENTLY IMPROVE YOUR WILLPOWER

While mindful awareness is the foundation of your new, healthier relationship with alcohol, another key element is, of course, willpower. Unfortunately, we are constantly bombarded with advertisements, marketing, native content, must-haves and an endless ocean of stuff that we have to use self-control to ignore. We are relentlessly seduced into feeling discontent with what we have, and this discontentment is the biggest challenge to our willpower.

Many psychologists believe that willpower is like a muscle, which has its downsides (it gets tired) as well as its upsides (it can get stronger). This is why our self-restraint is lower at the end of the day when we find it more difficult to make healthy decisions. Decision fatigue is the reason why some hugely successful people (notably Barack Obama, Mark Zuckerberg and the late Steve Jobs) wear the same thing every single day. It frees up their brains for the important decisions. Marketers are all over decision fatigue – they bloody love it. It leads to impulse buying, and it's the reason why so many people can't resist the treats at the checkout after a decision-heavy trip around the supermarket. Yes, making too many decisions leads to a lack of self-control. This is also known as ego-depletion. So, as far as you can, try to limit unnecessary decisions in your life.

Another form of decision fatigue is analysis paralysis, whereby a person overthinks (and therefore, overcomplicates) a situation to the extent that they end up not doing anything about it. Sound familiar? If you've ever found yourself standing in Pret staring at the sandwiches, frozen with indecision, that's the same analysis paralysis that has you knocking back that glass of wine just because it's there. To me, this is epitomised by attempting to drink less but getting so caught up in how to do it that I end up thinking, fuck it, and having a glass of wine anyway.

The main reason many people find abstaining from alcohol entirely to be easier than moderating their drinking is precisely because they have made one decision: I don't drink, ever. This eliminates the need for hundreds of other decisions. Should I drink tonight? How much? What shall I drink? What do I say when someone offers me a drink? How can I avoid being coerced into drinking more than I want to?

You probably didn't realise quite how big a role the science of decision-making plays in the strength of your willpower. People think that if they give in to the offer of an alcoholic drink on a day when they had intended to be alcohol-free, that means they are weak or lacking in self-control. This is absolutely not the case. It simply means that we were unprepared and made a snap decision without really thinking about it. Or at least only thinking about it in the unconscious part of our brain, which has been programmed over a lifetime to believe that alcohol is a vital part of a fun night out. Those snap decisions have nothing to do with logic or rational thinking.

This is also the reason why people who think they have excellent self-restraint often fail at moderate drinking, because they believe that determination alone will get them through it, and they don't create structures (such as goal-setting, planning and mindfulness) to support them to make more conscious decisions. This was always my downfall.

We're going to build those structures now and, once in place, you'll find that moderate drinking is not only possible, but actually exhilarating and empowering.

NOTES

4

THE PLAN

You have acknowledged the problem, and learnt to stop blaming yourself for the over-drinking that has been a deeply ingrained part of your life until now. You've read the incentive, and feel committed to a more mindful relationship with alcohol, and you've prepared yourself mentally for the road ahead. Now I'm going to take you through the tools and techniques that have revolutionised the way that I drink (and, often, don't drink).

MEASURE AND MONITOR

Before you start trying to cut down, it's important to calculate exactly how much you drink in a standard week. The Department of Health's most recent alcohol guidelines in the UK recommend that both men and women drink no more than 14 units of alcohol a week. That's about six pints of beer or seven standard (175ml) glasses of wine.

When I realised I was having closer to 30 units every week – and on a particularly stressy or sociable week, it could be closer to 40 – I was shocked. The thing is, we compare our drinking not to the national average, but to those around us. Our friends and family. It might feel as if you don't drink much in the pub after work because Julia from HR is always sloshed. Or you might think a couple of glasses of wine every evening don't matter because your husband always polishes off the rest of the bottle, so at least you're not having *that* much.

Working out exactly how much you're drinking can be tricky because 'a glass of wine' can be a variety of sizes, and that craft beer often has a stronger ABV (alcohol by volume) than a pint of lager. Luckily – as with everything these days – there's an app for that. Drinkaware has lots of online tools to help you work out exactly how much you drink, but most useful is the free app: Drinkaware Track and Calculate Units. You can tap to add drinks (do this as soon as you have them, so you don't forget how many you had) and you can even specify brands and measurements so the unit calculation is accurate.

Input every drink over the course of a week and you will have a picture of your drinking. Having this information will give you a chance to reflect on how much you drink, and work out exactly what a healthy relationship with alcohol means to you.

Tracking your drinking will not only show you the initial extent of the problem, but also research has shown that monitoring habits actually helps to improve them. This is why people who want to lose weight are often advised to keep a food diary, or people who want to spend less should keep a record of their spending. As well as simply monitoring your drinking, the Drinkaware app allows you to set specific goals, and be sent alerts and reminders to keep you on track. So keep it on your home screen – it's going to be useful throughout your 28-day Clean Break and while you reintroduce alcohol in a more moderate way.

There are oodles of other apps if, for example, you prefer a more stylish design (Drinks Meter) or you want something specifically for a sober month (Dry January & Beyond). And Club Soda's online community also has a weekly goal-setting and progress update tool.

David Crane, of UCL's Department of Behavioural Science and Health, devised the Drink Less app as part of his PhD. He and his colleagues were testing whether different behaviour-change techniques are more or less effective and, initially, they had two versions of the app. One was very basic: it prompted users to record their drinks every day but didn't give them much feedback other than a simple graph. The other version had every self-monitoring tool they could think of, so lots of graphs and analysis and feedback. Interestingly, both groups reduced their alcohol intake, but the difference between the two was negligible. 'What that shows is that self-monitoring itself is valuable and that the effects of self-monitoring can take place even when people don't really have the tools to do it,' says Crane. 'Even very simple monitoring or reflecting on your drinking can encourage you to moderate.' Why? 'Fundamentally what's happening is that people are becoming more aware of what they're doing,' he explains. 'They're not even necessarily more aware of its effects. Most people have a sense in their mind of what an acceptable level of drinking is, and they may be unconscious of that most of the time, and what self-monitoring does is it brings that to consciousness.' It all comes back to awareness.

If you prefer to limit the digital clutter in your life, and the number of apps on your home screen, use a good old notebook and pen. As David Crane pointed out, no method of monitoring is too basic, and there is evidence to show that the physical act of writing down a goal strengthens commitment (which is why, when it comes to goal-setting in the next section, I'm going to ask you to write things down with an actual pen). If you do decide to use a notebook, having extra space means that, unlike on the apps, you could also write down how you felt before and after drinking. This will help you be crystal clear about the reasons why you drink (for example, stress), and the imagined result (relaxation) versus the actual result (still stressed, but now hung-over, too). If you are able to monitor things like your mood, energy, weight, sleep or spending, you will begin to see really quantifiable improvements in your life, and that will inspire you to keep going.

I'm a fan of stationery porn, and I can spend hours leafing through lovely new notebooks and working out exactly how I'm going to format my ideas and plans inside them. My favourite form of procrastination is watching YouTube videos of bullet-journalling and habit-tracking and how to make the perfect to-do list. But for your clean break, all you really need is one of those mini desk calendars where you can tick off (or give yourself a gold star) for every alcohol-free day. Yes, I know, like a toddler's reward chart. Our brains are not all that different from toddlers' brains, really, and those charts exist because they work. *Everybody* loves getting a gold star.

TRY THIS

While one or two alcoholic drinks might make you a buzzier version of yourself, any more than that has the opposite effect. Try this trick on a night out to monitor the impact of your drinking. After every alcoholic drink, go to the loo and take a selfie. It's a failsafe way of proving that, while two drinks = sexily dishevelled, five drinks = smudged mascara, droopy eyelids and red-wine teeth. It's a highly effective wake-up call.

THE 28-DAY CLEAN BREAK

This book is about moderation, not abstinence. So why is a clean break so important? First of all, it marks the end of an unhealthy relationship with alcohol and the start of healthier one. It will give you an opportunity to see the problem. By that I mean the ways in which you had been relying on alcohol, or mindlessly drinking. And you need to be able to see the problem in order to be able to deal with it. If you want to reorganise your wardrobe, you can't simply have a quick browse through it, making instant decisions about what to keep. You have to take everything out, then only put back the things you really love. This is what we're going to do with your drinking.

When I started researching how to drink more moderately, the importance of a complete break from alcohol came up time and time again.

Laura Willoughby of Club Soda says they always recommend a break from drinking – what they call a 'sober sprint' – before attempting a new, moderate relationship with alcohol. 'The sprint will let you know what your key triggers are, and who the people are that might be your biggest pitfalls, so that when you come to plan your journey to moderation, you can work out how you're going to deal with those,' she explains.

So whether it's social drinking, a stress-numbing G&T after work or the routine of opening a bottle of wine at home every evening, this is your chance to identify your habitual behaviours.

Once ingrained, a habit is something you do automatically, without even thinking about it. That's what makes them so difficult to break. And for many of us, drinking has become habitual. How long does it take to break a habit? Well, the jury's out. The received wisdom is 21 days. A more recent study[24] said it's 66 days. Some people claim it's just three days. It depends on the individual, the severity of the addiction and timing. For our purposes, I propose 28 days. It's short enough to be manageable, but long enough to be tricky.

I took a break while I threw myself into the research and interviews that would teach me how to be a more mindful drinker. Like many people, I found it easier to abstain with a set period of time in mind. After four weeks, I felt better in every way: more energy, less anxiety and a better sleep pattern. I even found it easier to go to bed at a reasonable time, because I didn't feel compelled to stay up for one more glass of wine and one more episode of the latest Netflix drama.

Drinking increases your tolerance, so the more you drink, the more you need to drink in order to get the same effect. Resetting your tolerance will make moderation easier, as long as you approach it properly (which we'll come to later). Attempting moderation with no plan will see your drinking escalate back to

24 Cancer Research UK Health, Behaviour Research Centre, 2009

normal levels just as fast as mine did post-pregnancy.

Your long-term moderate drinking success will benefit hugely from immediate tangible results. Nobody wants to persevere with something they feel isn't actually doing them any good. But after just one month alcohol-free, you should already be enjoying more energy, more restorative sleep, clearer eyes and skin, a sharper brain at work and more money in the bank. Depending on your lifestyle (i.e. assuming you haven't replaced alcohol with cake) you will already be slimmer, too. The instant effects will inspire and empower you to change your relationship with alcohol forever.

Take this time to think carefully about the reasons why you want to cut down, which could be anything from weight loss to better sleep, from saving money to being more productive at work. Or maybe it's about your relationships, and being a better and more present partner, parent or friend. This is why you are going to reset your relationship with alcohol.

TIMING

Four weeks is a comparatively long time, so it's a good idea to think carefully about which month you choose to do your clean break. Don't tackle it in the month of your best friend's wedding or your summer holiday. If you can, aim for January or October, when there are already lots of people doing Dry January and

Go Sober October (or Octsober, which I strongly feel does not work as a portmanteau, but don't let that put you off). These campaigns are a great opportunity to take a break at a time when you'll be met with less social resistance. If you tell people you have decided not to drink for a month, that will probably bring up lots of questions, and perhaps some of your friends will even try to tempt you out of it. Whereas if you say, 'I'm doing Dry January', that's generally just accepted. You'll probably know other people who are doing the same thing, so there will be a level of social support, and you can share ideas about what you're drinking instead, or what you're doing in the evenings. Having that sense of community is an enormous help.

Having said that, part of the purpose of this clean break is to shatter your unhelpful ingrained beliefs that you need alcohol to have fun. So while I want you to go easy on yourself, I don't want you to stay in and watch boxsets for four weeks (although that brings its own sobriety challenges). During my clean break, I went out to a work event at which I could never previously have imagined declining a glass of wine, and I realised that having a sparkling water in my hand made no difference whatsoever. I had fun, and I felt a weird elation at the freedom of not having to think about my next drink, or if I was verging on having had too much. It was refreshing. I want you to get out and see people and realise that you can spend an evening with friends or colleagues and have a brilliant night, without any of the morning-after fatigue or anxiety.

FIND A SIGNATURE SOFT DRINK

Do not underestimate how important this part of the process is. You might think the main issue here is resisting an alcoholic drink, and a section on soft drinks is nothing more than super-fluous filler, but this step is vital because once you have found an alcohol-free drink that you enjoy and feel comfortable order-ing, you will never again panic, flail around and agree to a wine when someone else is getting a round in. Exploring the world of alcohol-free drinks is a great way to get through a month of sobriety.

Happily, avoiding alcohol no longer means sadly sipping a tepid, watered-down orange juice or an enamel-dissolving Diet Coke. Now there are a whole host of soft (or, to give them the drinks industry buzz word: 'zero-proof') drinks good enough to actually make you want to forsake that G&T. Drinks brands are cottoning on to the fact that younger people are drinking less than ever, and now a third of people in London and 20 per cent nationwide are teetotal.[25] That's a huge market of people who don't necessarily want to have to stick to water through lack of other options.

Victoria Moore is the *Telegraph*'s wine correspondent and author of *The Wine Dine Dictionary*, who has successfully

25 ONS

moderated her drinking over the past few years (particularly impressive in her line of work). As a result, her expertise has extended to 'grown-up' sophisticated drinks with no alcohol. She says botanical brewing is a big trend in zero-proof drinks. 'It simply means a substance that comes from a plant, so it could be peel, juice, root, leaf, bark, seed or flower,' she explains. 'Essentially, it's a more romantic way of saying that a drink has natural flavourings.'

One of the best-known brands in this area is Seedlip, marketed as 'the world's first non-alcoholic distilled spirit', infused with allspice and cardamom and served on ice with tonic. I have tried it and can confirm that not only is it delicious, but with its bouquet of natural infusions and no added sugar, it tastes like a properly grown-up drink. Which is refreshing when so many soft drinks make you feel like you should be sitting at the kids' table.

So the non-alcoholic gin gets my vote, but what about beers and wines (anything with less than 0.5 per cent ABV is considered alcohol-free, and below 1.2 per cent can be branded 'low-alcohol'). For many people, these drinks solve the problem of breaking a habit, because it requires very little behaviour change. You can still stand in the pub with a beer in your hand. If the ritual of opening a beer marks the transition to your downtime, find an alcohol-free version that you love and stock up on it. This is known as: 'keep the routine, change the substance'. It's the placebo effect, and it can be really powerful.

Among the most popular alcohol-free beers are Innis &

Gunn's Innis & None, St Peter's Without, Nirvana's Tantra Pale Ale and Brewdog's Nanny State. However, some people feel that a booze-free version of an alcoholic drink only makes them more keenly aware of what they're missing out on. And Moore tells me that 'alcohol-free wines are a complete waste of time and money.'

The good news is that there is now a whole new world of craft sodas that have been created not as a 'substitute' to alcohol, or something that is second best, but as a delicious and aspirational choice. Hunt down Kitsch Drinks, Square Root, Steep Soda, Karma Cola, Soda Folk, Dalston's, Nix & Kix, Ugly and Shrb – all cool craft brands with a focus on style *and* substance.

Mustafa Mahmud is the founder of Shrb, a botanically brewed 'prohibition soda'. The original 'shrub' was created in eighteenth-century England where, after preserving fruit people would drink the fruity vinegar. In America, shrub thrived during prohibition thanks to the vinegar kick that made it a more sophisticated choice than a sugary soda. 'We steep our ingredients in apple cider vinegar, which is like the distilling process because it releases all of the flavours without damaging them,' Mahmud explains. 'So you end up with a drink that is very low in sugar, and has a bite to it.'

An important aspect of Shrb's success – it is stocked in trendy craft breweries and places like Daylesford Organic – is that the design and packaging are stylish. 'If you buy cornflakes or healthy food, it goes into your cupboard at home, but a drink is one thing that is visible,' says Mahmud. 'You're holding it in your hand when talking to people. It says something about you. It's part of your identity.' And the fact that the bottle in your hand needn't be an alcoholic drink is all part of a wider cultural change. 'I don't drink, and in the past, I would have been in the pub with colleagues with a J20 in my hand. Not cool,' laughs Mahmud. 'But now I feel this social change is happening. It's about treating people like grown-ups and not talking down to them. Don't shout at people about your drink being low-sugar or alcohol-free. It is what it is. If you like it, drink it.'

And don't forget about hot drinks on your go-to list. What's Victoria Moore's favourite alcohol-free drink? 'If I'm honest, it's probably tea,' she says. 'I pretty much run on Yorkshire teabags. But I also love to take the time to make a pot of fresh white, green or black tea. The fragrance and provenance can be just as intoxicating and interesting as that of a good wine.'

....

WHAT TO ORDER DURING YOUR CLEAN BREAK

- The recent enormous popularity of gin means there has been a parallel surge in delicious high-end tonics. Try Fentimans, Fever Tree and good old Schweppes Indian Tonic. One of those with a slice of lime looks just like a G&T and is delicious.
- I used to say brunch isn't brunch without a Bloody Mary. Now, unless it's a special occasion, I go for a just-as-delicious and way-more-virtuous Virgin Mary. Just make sure they don't

scrimp on the Tabasco so that you get that kick.

- Bitters are great for solving the issue of so many alcohol-free drinks being sickly sweet (I mean, what's the point of not drinking if you're going to feel like throwing up in the taxi home anyway?). A soda water with a dash of Angostura bitters hits the spot.

- Kombucha is made with 'live' fermented tea, so it's packed with nutrients and great for your gut. Search out craft kombucha brewers like Equinox, Love, Jarr, or Profusion, whose kombucha is available from Ocado.

- If a bar has a cocktail list, it will almost certainly have an alcohol-free section. If not, just ask. Mixologists love showing off, so they'll relish the challenge of creating something bespoke.

- For widely available botanically brewed deliciousness, try Folkington's, Belvoir, Luscombe and Peter Spanton.

- A bitter lemon is a great option, assuming you don't mind (or perhaps you quite enjoy) the slight vibe of Dot and Ethel in the Queen Vic. Personally, I love a bit of 1970s kitsch, and a bitter lemon is usually served on ice in a low-ball glass, so it is perfect for evenings when you don't want to make a big deal of not drinking, because it looks like a 'proper' drink.

LEARNING SOBER SOCIALISING

While it might sound, and initially feel, incredibly weird to 'learn' sober socialising, that's what you have to do, because so many of us have never, ever done it.

I gave up drinking briefly in my first year of university. The main reasons were money and vanity because, after six months of beer and cheesy chips, I felt fat, lethargic and broke as a joke. I remember it was a revelation to dance sober in the student union and turn up to a lecture without a hangover. Why was I so unself-conscious? Maybe because I was 18 years old, so excited to have moved to London and gleefully realising that not drinking meant I could splurge more of my student loan in Topshop. I can't remember why I started drinking again (it probably involved a boy), but this unlikely alcohol-free period of my university life only lasted a few weeks. The fact that I did it then means I know I can do it now.

There are several techniques you can use to help you get the hang of sober socialising. A key one is to take the focus off yourself and put all your attention on others. This makes you feel less self-conscious, because you will realise that everyone else has their own shit going on. And it makes you a better friend/colleague/partner because you will be able to really listen to what the other person is saying and respond with interest and compassion.

Sobriety requires creativity, so think about what you love. Perhaps you could get into outdoor film screenings, or late-night museum and gallery openings, or ice-skating, or ten pin bowling, or going on long walks. Perhaps you could rope a friend into doing some kind of evening class with you – cooking or dancing or pottery.

Without alcohol, it's really only possible to have fun with people who genuinely lift your spirits, so your clean break might make you reassess some of your friendships. If you can't enjoy a person's company without booze, is it really such a great loss if you see less of that person?

Then it's about learning to be OK with the fact that your social life might now look a little bit different. 'If the fact that you're not drinking means that you can't stay up until 4 o'clock in the morning talking crap and solving the world's problems, that's fine,' says Lauren Booker of Alcohol Concern. 'It's OK to say, "actually, it's midnight and I'm knackered. I'm going to bed now."'

Hmm ... surely easier said than done, because your friends might roll their eyes or wonder what happened to the party girl that used to be the last one standing?

'It's all about our own perception,' explains Booker. 'Switch it around. If we've got a friend who says they feel like an early night, we'd be fine with it. We do it to ourselves. We feel that we have to justify it because alcohol has become so ingrained. But actually, the longer you are moderate or abstinent, the more people you will find come up to you and ask how you are doing it. People come out of the woodwork and tell you that they're impressed with what you're doing and they want to try it as well.'

Social proof is the psychological phenomenon of seeing other people, just like you, behaving in a certain way. So the more you do sober socialising, the more others in your social group will see there are plenty of options other than drinking, and they will want to get involved.

Supporting others actually helps you, too. In the same way as they say that the quickest way to be happy is make someone else happy, supporting others will help you feel more supported. Seek someone else who wants to moderate their drinking and put effort into helping them.

I want you to forget the perceived stigma of not drinking and throw yourself fully into sober socialising during your clean break. Once you've done that, you'll know you can, which will make moderation so much easier.

....

TRY THIS

Be generous. When out for dinner with friends, split the bill equally, regardless of how much wine they had that you didn't. It's likely that if one of the group isn't drinking, the others will drink less anyway, so the bill will be cheaper overall. And your bill is

PREPARE FOR YOUR CLEAN BREAK

Take some time to think about what will motivate you this month. This is an opportunity to reevaluate other parts of your life. Are you happy with your work life, your relationships, your social life, your body? If you've always loved dancing but couldn't imagine doing it without drinking, you could sign up for that after-work Beyoncé dance class that you always wanted to try. If you're more of a morning person, make the most of your new hangover-free mornings by doing an early yoga or spin class. If you've always wanted to write a book or start your own business, now could be the time to take the class or do the work that is going to make that possible. Once you start to focus on the things that are important, with all the renewed energy and productivity that you have gained through drinking less, your reinvention will happen naturally. And the new you will be far more authentic because she is no longer being numbed or blocked out by booze.

Being free from alcohol can drive hugely positive personal change, and having a parallel challenge can be a really strong incentive to stick with sobriety. But – and this is a big but – make sure you're throwing yourself into something that you're going to love, because otherwise you could become overwhelmed and simply give up.

'If it's hard for you to give up drinking, you might not want to ask too much of yourself', agrees happiness and good-habits guru Gretchen Rubin. 'Like, if you want to train for the marathon, think about the fact that you haven't been running in five years. If you're giving up drinking at the same time, maybe you're setting yourself up for feeling that you can't handle it. It's important to be realistic because sometimes people think, "I'm going to turn over a new leaf and this new, exciting person is going to spring out of bed and quit drinking and train for the marathon!" But you're still the old you. So it *could* be an exciting time to do that, but I could see it going both ways.'

Personally, I found it inspiring and galvanising to have the parallel challenge of writing this book alongside my clean break. But perhaps you need to be gentler with yourself this month, and not pile additional challenges on top of not drinking. Everyone's different, so it's a matter of working out what's most motivating for you, to give you the best chance of succeeding.

One thing that's motivating for everyone is a reward. Arguably, waking up clear-headed and knowing that you didn't leave your credit card behind the bar and your phone in the taxi is enough of a reward, but it's good to have something else to look forward to. Work out how much money you'll save over a month of not drinking and plan to use that for a massage or other treatment at the end of the month. Or break down your month into weekly rewards, for example, a delicious Sunday brunch, with the added bonus of no hangover.

'Healthy treats are important,' agrees Rubin. 'A massage is good. Or make plans with a friend you haven't seen in a long time. Maybe let yourself download some trashy television or re-read a book that you love. I would be careful about replacing drink with food, because you don't want to go from alcohol to sugar. That's very easy to do because you might think, "I just ate 30 cookies but at least I'm not drinking."'

Working out what constitutes a booze-free reward for you is actually quite fun. For so many years, a glass of wine was my 'treat' at the end of the day. Now I've realised that – with my hectic job, family and social life – a treat for me is actually just to lie on the sofa, listening to a podcast and staring into space. Bliss.

Fighting your cravings, working out rewards and motivating yourself is only part of what it takes to get through a month of sobriety. It gets more complicated once other people come into play. Think carefully about potential pitfalls. It is so easy to fall back into drinking, because that has been our standard habit and response for so long. Sticking to your month off will take some thought, effort and preparation. It's vital to take an organised approach, identifying a plan for every potential pitfall, so you never find yourself having to make a decision about whether or not to drink on the spot. Always have a soft drink on the tip of your tongue, and a back-up plan if they don't have what you want (everywhere has lime and soda).

Take some time to anticipate who you're going to see tonight and whether anyone will be uncomfortable with you not drinking, or might even try to bully you into it. I would never recommend not going out, because sociability is a vital part of a happy life, but perhaps you need to slightly rethink your social situations for the time being if you foresee issues. Will there be some element of the evening that you can focus on rather than booze, i.e. food, theatre, music? Are you going to be upfront about not drinking, and will a simple 'I'm not drinking tonight' suffice or do you need to have a planned excuse? Remember, you don't have to justify yourself to anyone, but it's worth thinking ahead to make life easier.

Ask yourself, too: are you looking forward to it? A night out with good friends is something to be cherished whether you're drinking or not. Think about why you enjoy being with them, what you want to talk about or hear about from them. If you're going out with people you merely tolerate rather than actually like, maybe just don't bother. If you do decide to go (and it's never compulsory) always plan your exit strategy in advance.

You can do this. The fact that you have committed time and money to buying this book shows that you are ready. Now let's look at some potential danger zones.

DRINKING DANGER ZONE 1:
THE AFTER-WORK PUB

If you can bear it, tell as many of your colleagues as possible that you are not drinking for one month. The more people in the office who know about it, the less likely they are to try to twist your arm and make you have a glass of wine. If you don't want to go into the details of your Clean Break with Simon from IT, it's a good idea to have a list of excuses up your sleeve:

- 'I overdid it last night and can't face a drink.'
- 'I've got an early meeting tomorrow.'
- 'I'm doing Dukan/Atkins/5:2.'
- Or, my personal favourite, brightly announce: 'I'm pregnant!' Then have a right old laugh at their shocked face.

If you don't want to make a thing of it by telling people that you're not drinking, buy your own first drink so you don't get involved in rounds, and make it something like a tonic, which looks like an alcoholic drink anyway. Flit around, chatting to different people, and every time someone offers you a drink, just nod to your tonic and say, 'got one, thanks'. The more drunk your colleagues become, the easier it will be for you to perform a 'French exit'. No, it's not a sex act, it's the art of leaving a social occasion without saying goodbye to anyone. They'll either think you did say goodbye and they've forgotten, or they were in the toilet when you left. Believe me, nobody will be offended. It's the quickest and easiest way to leave a boozy event.

DRINKING DANGER ZONE 2: AT HOME

Your approach to this danger zone will be different depending on who you live with, because the person or people with whom you share your home – if anyone – might be a big part of the reason why you drink. You might have a partner or housemate who loves to drink, but doesn't love to drink alone. You might have a child who – as much as you love them – drives you to exasperated exhaustion, so that opening a bottle of wine has become the thing you look forward to as soon as they're in bed. Or you might live alone and a drink with dinner has slowly but surely become a daily habit. So while drinking at home usually doesn't involve the social pressures of a night in the pub, it can be just as difficult.

Plan some strategies to deal with any cravings or desires for a glass of wine as soon as they come up. 'It's what we call dealing with discomfort, or "surfing the urge",' says Laura Willoughby of Club Soda. 'Your brain is like a petulant child. It will say, "I've had a hard day so I deserve it" and another part of your brain will say "but your goal is to be alcohol-free today", and it will escalate. So what you need to do is break that internal dialogue very quickly with a strategy. Whether it's walking around the block, doing some press-ups, cooking something nice, grabbing an alcohol-free drink from the fridge ... The minute that urge hits, if you can break that cycle with something else, the more likely you are to succeed.'

We'll go through many more distraction strategies and alternative ways to relax in the next chapter, and it's a good idea to have a list that you can refer to whenever you need to.

....

TRY THIS

Brush your teeth immediately after dinner. You're less likely to fancy a drink when you have a minty-fresh mouth (this technique also works if you're trying to stop pre-bedtime snacking).

....

DRINKING DANGER ZONE 3: A DATE

Back in my dating days, I used to say that I didn't trust a man who didn't drink. I would assume he had some kind of problem with booze. I'd think of our alcohol-free future together, with no glass of champagne in his hand at our wedding, and no wine with dinner ever again, and decide that this man would clearly not be my life partner. However, most of my dates started with me getting drunk too quickly because of nerves and ended with, let's just say, me not being my 'best self'. This is especially a problem here in the UK where, unlike other countries where couples have a series of civilised dates before taking their relationship further, we tend to drunkenly fall into bed together and only then try to work out if we like each other.

If you think it about it rationally, obviously a person who is capable of moderating their alcohol intake is going to be a better partner, a better lover, a better friend, a better parent and just a better person to have in your life. So be that person who orders a sparkling water, admitting you don't normally drink that much. I bet your date will breathe a sigh of relief that they don't have to get hammered, and you can find out if you actually like each other much more quickly, and with your dignity intact.

TRY THIS

Take a minute every morning to scan your plans for the day and anticipate any potential pitfalls. Who are you going to see? Do you have a work lunch or evening event at which drinks will be served? Are you out tonight, or in on your own? Just thinking it through will help strengthen your plan of action.

DRINKING DANGER ZONE 4: DINNER PARTY

This is a tricky one, because you're in a relaxed environment with friends. Generally everyone is drinking, and you're all sitting down together so everyone can see if you're not. There is no queue for the bar, and your glass seems to be magically topped up every time you take a sip.

Hopefully you have a good enough relationship with whoever is throwing the dinner party that you can explain to them that you're having a month off the booze. This is easier if it's Dry January or Sober October, but if not, you can say that you're not drinking for a month before your beach holiday, or you're having a break before the Christmas party season kicks in. If you drive, that's a good way to avoid drinking without making a thing of it because 'I'm driving' requires no more explanation as a reason not to drink.

The important thing is to tell your host in advance, so they don't seem disappointed when you refuse their carefully planned cocktail or glass of fizz on arrival. And do bring something with you that you're going to enjoy drinking – be that a nice bottle of Badoit or a selection of craft sodas – so the host has no sense of guilt that you're sitting there sipping a glass of tap water.

And (this is important) bring your dinner-party guest A-game. You have to prove to them that you are just as funny and interesting when you're not drinking as when you are. And the fact is, you *are* – you just haven't realised it yet. Focus on all the ways in which you are a better guest when you are not drinking. You will be capable of really listening when your friend tells you what's going on in her life at the moment, and offering advice with empathy and clarity. Your brain will be sharper and less fuzzy, so you'll be quicker with the jokes and anecdotes. You'll be particularly effusive about how delicious the food is, because you don't feel full and queasy from drinking. And you'll be able to read the cues when the host would quite like the guests to leave now, rather than drunkenly outstaying your welcome.

....

TRY THIS

Everyone has a friend that they only ever see at events where they are both completely hammered. Drop her a text and see if she's around for brunch at the weekend, or a coffee in the afternoon. Sober socialising skills are like anything else: they take practice. The more you arrange sober dates with friends, the less weird it will feel.

....

DRINKING DANGER ZONE 5:
DIFFICULT EMOTIONS

Whether you've been sideswiped by bad news, or are having a work or relationships-related personal crisis, it can take every last scrap of your self-control not to reach for the bottle. The key is to identify exactly how you are feeling and why. This is where mindfulness comes in again, because it's about awareness and taking time to check in with yourself.

Drinking to escape a negative emotion is *never* a good idea, because whatever it is will still be there the next day, just with the added complication of a hangover. Instead, identify a close friend or family member that you can call to talk your problem through with, and make sure they know that you are counting on them to get you through a rocky patch. They'll feel honoured that you trust them with such a responsibility and will do everything they can to help you.

If you are drinking in order to numb a feeling – be that stress, loneliness, boredom or anxiety – please remember that it's impossible to selectively numb emotions. Yes, you might temporarily block out whichever feeling you want to get rid of in that moment, but drinking will also block out your ability to feel happiness, love, gratitude, excitement and empathy. As one of my favourite writers, Brené Brown (known for her work on vulnerability and shame), says: 'Numb the dark and you numb the light.'

DRINKING DANGER ZONE 6: A WEDDING

As someone who attended several weddings during those tricky first three months of pregnancy when you're not supposed to tell anyone you're having a baby, I can tell you this is actually one of the easiest places to avoid drinking. Everyone gets so drunk so quickly that nobody really notices or cares if you're not drinking. Just grab a glass of fizz and hold it like a prop. No one will even notice that you're not drinking it. Job done.

A LAST WORD ON YOUR 28-DAY CHALLENGE

It's easy to feel zealous about the decision that has led to you feeling so much better in so many areas of your life. But when it comes to socialising, please don't make a big deal out of your decision to drink less. First of all, others may feel judged if they continue to drink. And secondly, it's like the old joke: have you heard the one about the vegan? Of course you have, because they tell you about it over and over and over again. Nobody likes hearing someone self-importantly bore on about their eating or drinking habits, and you attempting to convert a drinker to your moderation paradise is as tiresome as them trying to convince you to have a drink. At times like this, I call on the wisdom of Amy Poehler, who has a stock phrase that she uses when anyone proclaims the value of their own choices (whether in relation to parenting, drinking, or anything else). She simply says: 'Good for you. Not for me.' It's a brilliant line, which is both a celebration of difference and a firm assertion that you're sticking with what works for you.

The other important thing to bear in mind for your clean break is don't write it all off if you miss a day. You're not actually in AA. Nobody is going to ask you how many days sober you are. If you feel you have 'wasted' effort and willpower to get through, say, 25 days and then fail to make it to the end, that's just going to kill your motivation. Change your mindset completely: you went 25 days without an alcoholic drink – good work! Then take a moment to reflect on what caused the blip. It doesn't matter that you missed a day, what really matters is that you learn from it. Just try to do a few more drink-free days before moving on to the next step.

However, if after 28 days you feel so good about not drinking – with your improved sleep, clearer skin and more stable moods – that you want to carry on for a bit longer, please do. Your alcohol-free period is so important in your journey towards achieving moderation that, the longer you can do it, the stronger the foundations of your new moderate drinking life.

CLEAN BREAK CHECKLIST

- Find a signature soft drink.
- Spend a few minutes each day planning ahead for potential pitfalls.
- Learn to manage the discomfort of wanting a drink at home, and find something to distract you.
- Don't bore on about it to friends who are drinking.
- Reframe slip-ups in a positive way: i.e. now you've identified a trigger you can anticipate it in the future.

TRY THIS

I have a reminder in my phone that pings at 8 p.m. every night, telling me to update my drink-monitoring app. This is usually the time at which I'm thinking about a glass of wine, but the satisfaction of chalking up another alcohol-free day is the push I need to resist one.

MANAGE AND MAINTAIN

So you have completed an alcohol-free month. Well done! How do you feel? Are you already seeing and feeling some of the benefits? Was it harder than you thought, or easier?

You might think that you've done the hard bit now, but this is a common mistake and the reason why most people slip back into bad habits. I have a friend who refers to the period after Dry January as 'Wet February', and normally drinks twice as much as before. This is very common.

'When people decide to have a month off drinking and do Dry January, for example, they have the best-laid plans to go back in February and drink in a different way,' says Georgia Foster, hypnotherapist and founder of the Drink Less Mind programme. 'But if they have a history of drinking in unhelpful ways – binge-drinking, or over-drinking – the brain automatically goes back to the default of what's familiar. So people need to create habits that make a change that becomes a learned behaviour, which the brain then deems as familiar.'

The human mind truly is an incredible thing, and once your brain is retrained, it will do the work for you.

To avoid backsliding, Lauren Booker of Alcohol Concern urges an entire change of mindset. 'Never look at your month off drinking as a month's deprivation,' she says. 'Look at it only in terms of the benefits you will get. By the end of the month, your skin is going to be clearer, you'll have more energy. It's an opportunity for renewed health and vigour. It should be almost with regret that you feel you can now go back to drinking. That will help to ease you into February with an attitude of not wanting to blow all of those positive benefits. Also, remember that your tolerance has been lowered by a month off alcohol.'

It's easy to procrastinate and think of reasons why now is not the best time to start moderate drinking; it'll be easier after such-and-such an event, or so-and-so's party. Let me be very clear about this: NOW is the best time to start moderate drinking. Don't put it off.

Yep, the work starts here and it's really worth it, because this is a change for life.

GOAL-SETTING

By setting your goal I don't simply mean your goal of drinking less, I mean the goal of what you want to *achieve* by drinking less. Think about the effects of alcohol that we talked about in The Incentive, and identify which of those you would most like to address or remove from your life. What is most important to you?

Do you want to lose weight? Improve your skin? Save money?

Do you want to have better sex, or better relationships with your friends or partner?

Do you want to be happier and less anxious?

Do you want to be the type of parent who has the energy to build the world's tallest Lego tower before breakfast on a Sunday? (Or the patience to deal calmly with a tantrum.)

Do you want to be more productive at work? Or have the energy to take a leap at your long-held ambition of learning a new language, writing a novel or starting your own business?

Maybe you want improved sleep, or improved digestion. Or perhaps your goals are more about long-term health. Do you want to stick around to see your children grow up and to meet your grandchildren? Do you want to avoid the cardiovascular issues, liver disease or cancer within your family history?

Yeah, I know, there are so many benefits of drinking less alcohol that it's hard to whittle it down. But some of these must appeal to you more than others, so, whatever your specific aims, write down your top five and make sure you word it in a positive way – i.e. 'be happier' rather than 'less depressed', or, 'have more confidence' rather than 'have less social anxiety'. This is your Mindful Drinking Motivation: stick it somewhere that you'll see it every day. That could be on your computer, on your fridge or in the pages of your diary.

PLAN YOUR MINDFUL DRINKING
MOTIVATION HERE

....

....

....

....

....

....

....

....

....

....

....

....

....

....

....

....

....

....

....

....

....

....

The next step is thinking very carefully about what, where, when and how much you intend to drink in the future. Aiming simply to 'drink less' is way too broad a goal. You need to be very specific in your ambition. I go by the Rule of Three; this means I only allow myself to drink on three days every week, and on the days I do drink, I have no more than three drinks. I find this system really works because I'm not depriving myself. And, with my top limit in mind, I usually drink significantly less than that. Once you start drinking moderately, you'll soon realise that three drinking days in a week is plenty, and three drinks can get you nicely squiffy.

Personally, I don't get too hung up on counting units. The apps and tools we went through as part of your clean break are useful to keep track of progress, but if I spend too much time worrying about units, it makes me want to rebel and drink more. In the same way that people who obsessively count calories often end up bingeing on cake because the whole sorry process becomes too much. I think of the amount I consume in terms of the number of drinks I have, so, depending on what I'm drinking, this could be fewer units one night and more the next. I don't obsess over how many units are in a larger-than-usual glass of champagne, or try to work out what ABV that glass of wine is. I simply know that, as long as I stick to my Rule of Three, I'm drinking far less than I ever used to, and that's good enough for me. So, after your clean break you could simply compare how much you drank this week to an average week before you began to moderate your alcohol intake, and keep trying to reduce it.

However, if you're the kind of person who gets giddy over metrics and likes to go deep into stats, feel free to really get into units. If it's going to help you, and tracking your alcohol only in terms of drinks feels too woolly, then absolutely, go for it.

My Rule of Three might not be right for everybody. You might feel that three drinks is too many, or that four alcohol-free days a week is not enough. You need to decide on a rule that works for *you*, and no one else. It's all about being very clear in your approach to moderate drinking. Making a plan and sticking to it, leaving no room for deviation.

James Morris is the director of The Alcohol Academy, a non-profit organisation that offers training and consultancy for alcohol harm reduction. After realising that heavy drinking had become a habit in his twenties, Morris gave up completely for eight years, before deciding to reintroduce alcohol in a moderate way. He has now been drinking moderately for seven years, without any sign that he might slip back into his old bingeing ways. Rules, he confirms, are vital.

'It has been found that the setting of clear limits is an important predictor of success,' he says. 'My rules were that I would stick to the guidelines and, if I felt I was becoming dependent again, I would stop.' And are there any specific instances now when he knows not to drink, for example, when stressed or anxious? 'Yes, pretty much those! Or any other periods of low mood. Using alcohol to de-stress or escape is not OK.'

Not drinking to numb negative emotions is one of the other rules that work alongside my Rule of Three. There are others, too: I don't drink on more than two consecutive days, so my three drinking days are never all in a row. And I never drink alone. This one is pretty easy for me because I don't live on my own, so I don't get tempted by that, and my problem area was always social drinking anyway.

When setting your own personal goals, think very specifically about your own triggers and build your rules around those. Bear in mind that alcohol-free days are important for making sure your tolerance levels do not creep back up, so do include these in your planning.

When making your rule, consider:
- How many alcohol-free days do you want to have each week?
- What is the maximum number of drinks or units you will allow yourself on one day?
- How will you keep track of how much you're drinking (i.e. an app, or a nice notebook)?
- Are there any situations in which you won't let yourself drink (for example, if you're stressed, or having dinner with a difficult friend or relative)?
- Do you have any off-limits drinks? (Mine is white wine, which I tend to drink too quickly, and which reminds me of my boozy twenties.)

WRITE YOUR RULE HERE

....
....
....
....
....
....
....
....
....
....
....
....
....
....
....
....
....
....
....
....
....
....
....
....

Share your rule with as many people as possible, but if you can't face that, at least share it with someone close to you – perhaps your partner or a good friend. This sets your intention, helps you commit and provides accountability, which is an enormous help when adhering to any kind of plan, and also gives you someone to talk to when you need a boost.

Then set your rules in concrete. Stick to them no matter what. Remember Gretchen Rubin's strategy of the planned exception, whereby you can very occasionally break your rule as long as you've thought it through in advance? Implement it sparingly and always in a way that is meticulously planned. Once you have reinvented yourself and become comfortable with discarding your old identity as the person who is always up for a drink, those occasions on which you do drink are not backslides, they are simply planned exceptions. The key to making this work is in the planning. If you don't plan to drink, don't. I don't care if it's your best friend's 40th or your ex-boyfriend's wedding, as soon as you allow unplanned exceptions to creep in, that feeling of failure will send you back to an unhelpful drinking pattern really quickly. You have to train yourself to drink less, and the more you drink, the more you need to drink. So it stands to reason that the less you drink, the less you need to drink. Once you reduce your intake, you really will feel satisfied (and a bit drunk) after just a couple of drinks. Do not jeopardise that sweet spot with a binge.

Once you have identified your triggers, come up with what psychologists call 'if . . . then . . .' strategies. For instance, you might think, 'IF I want a drink to relax after the kids are in bed, THEN I'll have a bath and read a book instead.' Or, 'IF I want a gin and tonic after a stressful day at work, THEN I'll refer to my list of Mindful Drinking Motivation to reset my intention.' That's just two 'if . . . then . . .' examples, and you're going to need a lot of them, so plan ahead with a list of distractions, and healthy ways to relax, at your fingertips.

12-WEEK EVALUATION

Once you have set your intention, established your goals and made your drinking rules, you're well on your way to a better relationship with alcohol. Now you need to put a reminder in your diary or phone for 12 weeks from now, to evaluate where you are with your drinking. When you get to that day, ask yourself: are you still monitoring how much you drink? Are you sticking to your rules? Are your rules still working for you, or do you need to tweak them? Are you making an effort to live more mindfully? Do you refer to your Mindful Drinking Motivation as often as you need to?

If it's all going great, give yourself a pat on the back and set another reminder for 12 weeks from now. If you've slipped back into old habits, reset your intention, remind yourself of your goals, recommit to your rules and, if necessary, take another clean break.

Once you feel you've really cracked it, you can check in every six months, or even once a year. But do make sure you check in, because it can be so easy to slide back into old behaviours, even after months of moderate drinking.

TRY THIS

If, despite all your preparation, you find yourself in an unanticipated drinking situation and put on the spot when offered a drink, just make sure you pause before you answer. Take a deep breath and remember: one of the most immediate effects of alcohol is that it dehydrates you. This causes headaches, dry skin and tiredness. If you actually think about it, you know you'd prefer a refreshing, hydrating drink, of course you do. This is an important step towards drinking mindfully.

Now you have your clear goal, and your specific set of rules, I'm going to give you tips and tools to help you stick to them and manage your drinking for the long term. This is what worked for me, so I know it can work for you. Once again, it's all about awareness. Keep up the tracking techniques that we used for your clean break so you're always conscious of exactly what you're drinking. I still input my alcohol intake for the day into an app, every single evening. It takes a second, and I can see at a glance how much I'm drinking and how many alcohol-free days I've had.

Continued reflection on your goals, and on the benefits of drinking less alcohol, has been shown to be a key motivator in moderating your drinking, so do take time to regularly refer back to your Mindful Drinking Motivation. Reflecting with clarity on the benefits of not drinking requires you to be very clear about your thoughts and emotions. This is why it's important to include some element of mindfulness practice into your daily life. Remember, you don't have to formally meditate if that doesn't work for you. There are many ways to be mindful.

OPPORTUNITIES FOR NON-MEDITATION MEDITATION

- Walking (no headphones, please, unless you're doing a guided mobile meditation)
- Cooking
- Gardening
- Playing a musical instrument
- Exercise: running, yoga or whatever works for you

- Brushing your teeth or washing your hands. Any daily task can be turned into a mini meditation if you use it to focus completely on what you're doing.
- Lying in bed just before or after sleep.

··

TRY THIS

Look for moments throughout the day when you can focus on one thing. It could be eating, having a bath, or walking home from the station. Making it a habit to consciously reflect on the present moment will slow down that whirring mind, and living more mindfully will make better choices about your drinking come naturally.

··

DRINK MORE CONSCIOUSLY

Of the many ways in which you can incorporate mindfulness into your life, food and drink is one of the easiest. Not only can you mindfully get more enjoyment out of a drink, but you can also be far more aware of your cravings.

Say you've decided that today is going to be an alcohol-free day. If you feel like a glass of wine, and you try to resist that feeling, it will get bigger and bigger and bigger until it's overwhelming. If you catch the craving, and notice it mindfully, the whole experience changes. You can think, 'I want a glass of wine. Why is that? I feel anxious about what happened at work today. I feel tired because I didn't sleep well last night.' Now that you've seen your feelings for what they are, you know that it's not really about the wine. And you know that anxiety and sleep are both negatively affected by drinking, so you might talk to your partner/flatmate/mum about how you feel, then go to bed early with a good book or a favourite podcast. Noticing your feelings can help you choose the option where you wake up refreshed, having talked about your work stress and had a good night's sleep, rather than the option where you drink the wine and fall asleep in front of *Gogglebox*. Simply being aware of a craving can rob it of its power. It's like a soap bubble: as soon as you touch it, it pops.

There is nothing wrong with feeling these urges. It would be impossible to get rid of them altogether anyway. What you *can* do, though, is change the way in which you respond to them. This technique works just as well for unhealthy foods as it does for drinking.

'It's where this cliché of "the moment" comes in,' says Rohan Gunatillake. 'You know that you're going to be feeling crap about it later, so if you have the awareness to feel it being crap in the moment, you're less likely to do it.'

Gretchen Rubin calls this the strategy of the 'future self'. I know that 'future Rosamund' is going to be pretty disappointed tomorrow if she wakes up with a hangover. It sounds crazy, but it helps. 'It's an imaginative form of outer accountability,' explains Rubin, 'and it's a really powerful framework for a lot of people.'

Then if there is a drinking occasion that you know you are really going to enjoy, go for it. But go for it with full awareness. Really relish the joyful aspect of it, and stop when you've had enough. Drinking mindfully will make you keenly aware of how quickly that tipsy rush dissipates. It's why mindfulness and moderation go hand in hand, because you are able to see clearly when it stops being fun.

....

ROHAN GUNATILLAKE'S MINDFUL DRINKING EXERCISE

'For a ritualised coffee meditation, mindfully spend five minutes with your drink. Really notice your coffee. The colour of it, the flavour, the heat. Focus only on your coffee. Make it special.

This exercise gives you the benefits of formal meditation, and you know exactly what to do so there is no sense of feeling that you might be doing it wrong. There is no wrong. You can do this practice any time you have a drink that isn't alcoholic. It's training a behaviour that is being aware of what you're drinking, and it takes the pressure off anything to do with alcohol.

Mindfulness is about becoming really aware of what's happening while it's happening. If you are able to do this at work with lots of things happening around you, that's quite a high level of practice. It's like scaffolding for your mind.'

....

FORMING HEALTHIER HABITS

The best way to break a bad habit is to replace it with a good one. If you don't, the hole left behind by your old habit will need to be filled by something, and it could be that your glass of wine creeps its way back in. Either that, or you might mindlessly replace it with another unhelpful habit, like eating crap food or dumbly scrolling through the holiday photos of people you barely know on Facebook.

The *Telegraph*'s wine correspondent, Victoria Moore, has moderated her own drinking over the past few years. 'Now I don't drink unless I know I'm going to really enjoy what's in the glass,' she says. 'And if I'm drinking for escapism's sake, I try to realise that, and do a half-hour YouTube yoga video instead.' Interestingly, Moore recently completed a postgraduate diploma in psychology, so she knows a thing or two about how the brain works. 'Pouring a "the evening has started" drink can become a deeply ingrained habit,' she explains. 'And the best way to break habits is to train your brain to form new pathways. So, if every time you think, "6pm! Gin and tonic!" you make yourself go out for a run or put on the kettle for a pot of silver needle tea instead, before long you'll be making the decision to do that subconsciously, and not taxing your willpower at all.'

Initially, it is about finding alternative activities to distract you from drinking, but ultimately you can look at this as an opportunity to establish the habits you want to become everyday behaviours in your life – whether that's exercise, meditation, cooking good food or simply giving yourself regular pedicures. Forming healthier habits is the key to breaking out of bad ones.

Shona Vertue is a personal trainer, yoga teacher and creator of the Vertue Method, and she is the queen of healthier habits.

'We have come to rely on alcohol as an acceptable means for relaxation,' she says. 'Sadly it's really just a numbing agent. Truthfully, relaxation is not a given skill, it's a practice that must be trained, and that is why I highly encourage the practices of meditation and yoga.'

If you're finding it hard to stick to new, healthier habits and ways of relaxing, remember to focus on why you're doing this. 'When giving up alcohol, it's easy to get stuck in thinking about what you're losing or missing, but stay focused on how much more you're obtaining,' says Vertue. 'More money, better health, improved relationships, better sex . . . did I mention money?'

So, to establish those healthy habits (and thus replace the bad ones) we need to focus on our incentives and commit to practising our new habits over and over again. Repetition is absolutely key. This is why I keep referring back to your Mindful Drinking Motivation (see page 121). If you have tried and failed to cut down in the past, you simply may not have repeated your non-drinking behaviour enough for it to stick.

....

TRY THIS

Drink less but drink better. Victoria Moore says: 'Picking wine is so much more fun when you're buying a bottle you're going to be excited about. So is opening it. I buy half bottles so as not to waste a good wine by not drinking it.'

....

TRY THIS

Don't feel bad about throwing alcohol away. It's that first fizz of champagne that feels so good, or the first sip of that ice-cold G&T. Once you're over the initial buzz, it is no more wasteful to pour the rest of it down the sink as it is to drink it.

....

REFRAMING

We've talked about the theory of willpower as a muscle, but there is another argument that we can access fresh reserves of willpower simply by reframing our thoughts.

If you feel that you're depriving yourself, your journey of moderation will seem like a relentless struggle. Reframing is all about a simple change of perspective that can alter your experience in a dramatic way. Studies have found that those people suffering nerves before a particular event, rather than attempting to calm down, benefitted hugely from reframing their anxiety as excitement.[26] This is called 'anxious reappraisal' and it works because it's less of a leap from anxious to excited than it is from anxious to calm, since anxiety and excitement are both aroused emotions.

Almost anything can be reframed in a positive way. Think of an annoying, boring job, like paying the gas bill. If you take one minute to think about it positively, it changes the whole experience. Imagine living without hot water, or central heating. You're so lucky to have gas in your home, installed by experts, and running smoothly in such a way that you rarely have to even think about it, and you have enough money to pay for it, and it's easy because you can just do it online. All of a sudden, a boring job becomes something that you can actually appreciate.

'People often drink to get through a difficult or boring evening,' says Laura Willoughby, 'but that can easily be reframed in a positive way. If a person tells me, "I have to drink at this event because it's all my husband's friends so it'll be boring." I ask them, why are you going to something that you don't even want to go to? And they'll say, "because it's important to him."

26 *The Atlantic,* 2016

So that's how you reframe it. You have an opportunity to make your partner feel supported and, once this event is reframed as a positive act that you're doing for someone else, it's no longer something to endure.'

Research has shown that focusing on the positive benefits of doing something is far more effective than dwelling on the negative effects of not doing it. So refer again to your list of Mindful Drinking Motivation from the beginning of this section for a reminder of why you're doing this.

Drinking less alcohol is not about deprivation or endless struggles with self-control. It's about realising that you can be free from the emotional pull of alcohol; learning exactly *why* you drink, and controlling the situation so that you only do so on your own terms – not because of habit or societal pressures. Feeling more positive now? If not, we need to get to work on your inner critic.

....

TRY THIS

Take the five Mindful Drinking Motivation aims you wrote down at the start of this section and film yourself on your phone reading them out. Then, if you're having a wobble when out with friends, pop to the loo and watch it (use your headphones to avoid being judged by the person in the next cubicle).

....

BEAT NEGATIVE SELF-TALK

'I'm less fun sober.'

'I don't have the willpower for this.'

'Everyone thinks I'm boring.'

'People are judging me for not drinking.'

'This'll never last.'

Everyone has that voice in the back of their mind. Psychologists call it the 'inner critic' and, as critics go, it's a particularly brutal one. Even if you manage to make meditation a regular practice, you will not be able to completely quieten your mind. Nobody can, because at any point there are dozens of thoughts, feelings, opinions, fears, decisions, emotions, desires, worries and ideas (and often contradictory ones) clambering around in your brain. With mindfulness, you will be more aware of what your mind is doing, although, initially you might not like it.

'If we talked to our friends the way we talk to ourselves, we wouldn't have any friends left,' says Andy Cope, a positive psychology expert and the author of *Happiness: Your Route-Map to Inner Joy*. Cope has been studying what he calls the 'Two Percenters' – the people who are the happiest and most positive 2 per cent of the population – to see what they do differently. 'They still have that inner voice, but they're more friendly with themselves,' he explains. 'If someone asks them about their day, they'll only share the highlights. That trains the brain to pick out the good stuff instead of the bad stuff.' He's quick to add that this doesn't come naturally. 'Everybody's default position is critical unless we put strategies in place to change that. We are preprogrammed to see danger, to spot enemies and problems. And, because happiness doesn't save your life, it just enhances it, we're not programmed to tune into it as much.'

It feels easier to forego giving yourself a positive pep talk in favour of focusing on getting through the week so that you can enjoy the ephemeral release of a drink on Friday night. I've been there. Changing long-held thought patterns takes conscious effort; you must mine your deepest levels of commitment and determination to make positivity and optimism stick. The trouble is, your brain may still believe the negative thought, even as you're trying hard to focus on the positive thought. Cope describes this feeling as 'like a civil war inside your head'. This is why it takes work. Some people find it easier than others, since some are genetically predisposed to being happier, in the same way that one might have a genetic tendency to be thinner. Either way, it takes effort to make the most of what we were born with.

'It's not an overnight process,' says Cope. 'If you want a six-pack stomach, you can't just go to the gym once. You have to go regularly and there will be effort involved. It's the same with happiness. If you stop using the positive mental habits (such as focusing only on the good things) then you will regress back into negative self-talk.'

A big part of the appeal of drinking is that it shuts down your inner critic. This sounds great in theory, but the alcohol is also shutting down those other voices in your head that are actually saying some pretty useful things, such as 'you've had enough', or 'don't send that text to your ex'.

Your inner critic and your inhibitions are two sides of the same coin. They're there to protect you. Self-doubt is no bad thing; it is this self-doubt and an anxiety about the outcome of something that compels you to focus on it, and it makes you study for that important exam, prepare for that big meeting and work to meet that tight deadline. I wouldn't have got this book written had I not been anxious that I'd miss the deadline. It's what made me switch off my phone and get on with it.

Unfortunately, though, the other thing your negative voice often does is give you an endless stream of excuses to drink:

'My friend will be offended if I don't drink at her party.'

'She's broken up with her boyfriend so needs me to get drunk with her.'

'Work deals are done over drinks and I'll miss out if I don't join in.'

Tune in to when that voice is giving you those excuses and re-alise that they are meaningless. There will always be an occasion when you feel you ought to drink; once you are able to recognise those thoughts, you can replace them with more helpful, positive ones. This is another area where mindfulness can help because you can learn to see your thoughts without acknowledging them to be true. Remember: thoughts are not facts. Often, simply acknowledging negative thoughts can rob them of their power.

The goal of mindfulness is not only to be aware of your thoughts, but also to look at them without judgement. That is easier said than done, of course. But the more time you spend paying mindful attention to your thoughts, the more you can learn to notice them without having any judgey feelings about them. The skill is to introduce generosity and kindness into the way that you talk to yourself, and that takes practice.

Rohan Gunatillake explains it like this: 'Through mindfulness, you'll be able to see your anxiety and your pattern of drinking, and you are probably able to observe that neutrally. The judgement that comes on top of that – that commentary and the inner critic – feels more real. It's harder to see that neutrally. But, with practice, the mind stops believing the default pattern that your thoughts about yourself are absolutely true. You might identify as an anxious person for years. And then you start doing meditation practice and you realise that, while there are some anxious thoughts, there are also thoughts of kindness, and space between the thoughts. Then you believe your original thought less. Your belief in this core idea that "I am an anxious person" gets undermined.'

Since bringing mindful consciousness into my life, I am now capable of identifying anxious thoughts and rationally deconstructing them, taking steps to address them directly. Doing this, rather than trying to drown my stress in a fishbowl-size glass of wine, means I'm less likely to feel overwhelmed by challenging situations. This awareness also helps undermine other unhelpful thoughts, such as the disempowering idea that I need alcohol for socialising or stress relief.

This process doesn't happen overnight, and even if you have been doing it for years, negative thoughts will absolutely still creep in. It takes a change of thinking to be able to notice them, and dismiss them.

TRY THIS

At a party, hold your glass in your non-dominant hand. It sounds ridiculous, but just the act of doing something a little bit unfamiliar will make you drink more slowly and, yes, more mindfully.

GRATITUDE

Boredom and loneliness can be huge triggers for drinking. They both represent a gap in our lives – whether real or perceived. For example, some parents are triggered to drink because they resent the fact that they no longer have their old freedoms, and some people who don't have kids drink because they might see being childfree as something 'lacking' in their lives.

One of the best ways to diminish that gap is with gratitude. I'm sure you've heard all about the power of gratitude. The simple act of writing down things for which you are grateful, ideally every day, is one of the most popular and successful ways to retrain your brain out of negative thought patterns. It stops you taking things for granted. Not only the big things, like friends and family, but the little things, too.

'Most people spend an inordinate amount of time moaning about what they haven't got,' says Andy Cope, author of *Happiness: Your Route-Map to Inner Joy.* 'If you write down ten things that you are grateful for but you take for granted, it's really interesting because health and relationships come towards the top, but then it's things like the NHS, or having a roof over your head, or central heating. Then you'll realise that you don't actually need much more than what's on that list. You can make your whole day better just by being grateful for getting out of bed in the morning. Once again, that requires a retraining of your brain, which takes conscious effort.'

Gratitude is significantly easier once you are able to focus on the present moment. While eating dinner with my kids, I used to have half an eye on them while looking at work emails on my phone, fretting about all the things I should be doing, or looking at an event on Instagram that I might have been at had I not had children, and thinking about the glass of wine I can have once they're in bed. As soon as I decided to focus fully on the kids while I'm with them (safe in the knowledge that I'll focus fully on work later) then I actually notice the silly song my son is singing or the way in which he surreptitiously tries to make his baby sister laugh by burping, and I can feel grateful for my kids, which replaces anxiety with joy. This is why mindfulness has gained traction within the field of positive psychology over the last few years.

'If you'd have asked me about mindfulness five years ago, I would probably have been a bit dismissive,' admits Cope. 'I don't meditate, but I am very much more mindful at times like when I'm out walking the dog. I can pick some blackberries and be in the moment. Once you learn to be more mindful, then the magnitude of the moment sinks in, and that can bring huge joy.'

Cope says one way of learning to appreciate the present moment is the strategy of '4,000 weeks'.

'That's the average lifespan,' he says. 'When you tell people they've only got 4,000 weeks, you can see them thinking, "shit, that's not long". What it boils down to is that you're only going to get one life. You're only going to get one go at each moment. When you think of it like that, every moment becomes really important. How many moments have I missed out on because I've been so busy putting my happiness off until Friday?'

Anything that helps you become more aware of the present moment will help you become more mindful, which will transform your relationship with alcohol. Because once you realise the power of 'now' you won't want to waste any more moments feeling queasy and out-of-control when drunk, or hung-over the following day.

Work out what makes you happy. Focus on those things and be bloody grateful for them. It will make your life better, and make good intentions easier to stick to.

TRY THIS

Knowing you should do these practices is one thing; remembering to do them is another. Try pairing positive practices with a simple habit that you already do every day. For example, when brushing your teeth at night, think of five things for which you were grateful that day. When your computer makes that start-up 'ping' noise as you switch it on, count five deep breaths. As you repeat these behaviours, your brain will learn the pattern and do it automatically.

SLEEP

It's impossible to overstate the importance of sleep. Arianna Huffington wrote an entire book about how it changed her life.[27]

27 Arianna Huffington, *The Sleep Revolution*, WH Allen (2016)

You ideally need seven or eight hours a night, particularly if you want the clarity of mind to make better decisions and have strong impulse control: both of which are vital for moderating your drinking.

We know that alcohol disrupts your sleep cycles, denying you the deep, restorative level of sleep that makes you feel refreshed the next day. This is why you can end up in a vicious circle of alcohol making you tired, and being tired making you less capable of resisting a drink.

If you've been drinking for a long time, it could take a while for your body to readjust to a normal sleep pattern. Plus, cutting down might have left your thoughts and anxieties raging out of control at night-time. Please don't lose heart if change doesn't happen instantly. Your brain needs to learn, without the aid of a drink, how not to allow disruptive thoughts to crowd your mind right before sleep. Mindfulness will eventually give you control of your thoughts to the extent that you are aware of your anxiety about work, or money, or whatever it is, but you are capable of putting your mind elsewhere. If that sounds overwhelming, I get it. Taking your focus away from your anxieties feels like an impossibility. Using mindfulness to change your thoughts sounds like next-level shit; as if you need to have spent a week on a mountain top with a silent man in flowing robes to be able to have that kind of Jedi mind control, but actually, training your brain to focus on the positives is one of the core techniques of good old positive psychology.

'Instead of counting sheep, count your blessings,' says Andy Cope, simply. 'Run through your day and think about what you are grateful for. The classic positive psychology activity is to keep a pen and paper by your bed and write down three good things that have happened during the day. That's been clinically proven to quieten your mind.'

Getting into good wind-down habits can revolutionise your sleep – and this means strict rules about social media before bed. You already know it won't make your mind feel calm and rested; more likely, you'll see photos from a holiday that you wish you were on, or your ex's hot new partner, or an article about a terrifying or heartbreaking war or political situation. Just don't do it.

Many people feel like they have given so much of themselves to other people all day that they deserve to claw back some time. If you've been working hard at your job all day, or focusing on your kids until they're asleep, of course you want to capture a bit of time at the end of the day. For me, this used to mean a glass of wine. Now I know that drinking is a thief of time, it makes me more inclined to replace it with something more meaningful and restorative, like a conversation with someone I love, or relaxing in a bath, or reading a good book.

Do give yourself time for sleep habits to click into place. It won't happen instantly, but when it does it will make a dramatic improvement to so many aspects of your life. Not only to your mood and energy levels, but also to less-obvious things such as assertiveness, empathy, concentration and emotional intelligence. Following good sleep-hygiene habits will make your journey to moderate drinking significantly less bumpy.

....

SLEEP HYGIENE HABITS

- As much as possible, go to bed and get up at about the same time every day.
- Instigate a social media cut-off point and don't look at Twitter, Facebook or Instagram after that time.
- Same goes for work emails. You're not going to do anything about that stressy missive from a colleague at 11 p.m., so you might as well not see it until the morning.
- You know how they recommend a bedtime 'routine' for getting a child to sleep? Well, having a bath and reading a book will do the same for you as it does for a two-year-old.
- Having something that signals it's nearly time to sleep is a good way to programme your mind to wind down. Whether it's a cup of mint tea or a piece of relaxing music.
- Exercise. Don't pump iron right before bed or anything, but being a bit more active during the day will help you drop off at night.
- Invest in a blackout blind and make your room as dark and calm (i.e. uncluttered) as possible.
- Once you're in bed, find something either positive or neutral for your mind to focus on. Count your breaths in and out, up to ten, and then start over again. If your mind wanders, just

gently bring it back to your breath.

- If your mind is still whirring, try listening to a podcast, or there are many other relaxation and hypnotherapy downloads specifically designed to help you drop off.

- If you're feeling like 'just one drink' will help, remember that switching off your phone and having a bath will do the same job and won't wake you up with that 3 a.m. dread.

....

THE POWER OF VISUALISATION

You might have heard of visualisation as a technique that athletes use before a big sporting event. They literally imagine themselves doing a brilliant job at it and, unlikely as this sounds, doing so actually stimulates the relevant neurons in the brain, which has been proven to make them perform better. You can use the same technique before a big presentation or a job interview. Or you can use it as one of the tools to help you drink more moderately.

Think about the best possible version of yourself: it's you after an excellent night's sleep, at your sharpest and brightest, on your best hair (and skin) day ever. Does that person want a drink? Hell no. She doesn't need one. Imagine her happily chatting to friends while sober at a party, or working at an exciting side project on her laptop with a mint tea, or sinking into a relaxing bath after the kids are in bed. You can do this just before you fall asleep at night, or when you wake up in the morning. Picture every single detail of that person and keep her in mind when entering a 'drinking danger zone'.

You could also think of this process as 'rehearsing'. You already know that you need to prepare for anything at which you want to do well, so why would that be any different for not drinking? Rehearse in your mind exactly what you're going to say when offered a drink, or if your booziest friend tries to push you to have one, or if someone buys you one without asking, or if your favourite cocktail is on the menu, or if your friend tells you that the wine is organic so it won't give you a hangover ... Rehearse every eventuality and you'll be well prepared to go into the fray.

....

TRY THIS

Stick to drinks with which you're familiar. This helps you feel in control. If you've already decided you're only drinking gin and tonic, you're not being drawn into making a snap decision over the cocktail list, or accepting that ill-advised shot.

....

ALTERNATIVE STRESS-RELIEVERS AND CELEBRATIONS

One of the most common justifications we give ourselves for drinking after work is the old classic: 'I deserve it'. Whether you've had a great day, a terrible one, or even one that's simply mediocre; the reasons why you 'deserve' a drink are manifold: you had a great meeting, a really bad appraisal, you got that month's highest sales figures, or your sneaky colleague passed off your idea as his own and there's no way you can tell people without looking bitter and whiny.

Of course, there is absolutely nothing wrong with having a glass of fizz to celebrate a promotion, and enjoying a drink with a positive attitude can be great, but now that you know the link between alcohol and anxiety, you know that drinking to try to improve your mood is actually only going to plunge you into a vicious circle of low mood, heavy drinking and poor sleep.

'Once I had a stressful day at work and I was stomping around Soho thinking, this is when I would normally have a gin and tonic,' says Laura Willoughby of Club Soda. 'So instead I went into Boots and bought a really expensive beauty product. And that seemed to fill the same gap. That feeling of treating myself, of reward, of distraction. I managed to achieve it with that one act.'

Drinking at home can be a danger zone, particularly if you live alone. Now, I am not of the attitude that people who drink on their own have a problem. If you live on your own, it absolutely does not make you an alcoholic if you have a glass of wine with dinner. But I want you to enjoy a drink in a way that makes you happy and relaxed. Always be aware of *why* you are drinking, and if you are drinking your feelings, stop right now. Having someone else around – be that family, a housemate or a partner – can either help or hinder your journey of moderation, depending on that person. So it doesn't necessarily make you more likely to over-drink if you live on your own, but it is something of which you have to be wary, simply because there is no one there to judge you if you open a second bottle, or go to bed in the early hours. If this is your danger zone, it's a good idea to start some kind of project that doesn't involve drinking. Write in a journal. Learn how to give yourself a facial. Do a jigsaw. Organise your photos. Get one of those mindful colouring books. Meditate.

Regardless of whether you live alone or not, you need to find a way to quieten your mind without alcohol. So have a think about things that feel celebratory, or make you feel relaxed. I mean, sit down with a pen and paper (rather than a phone or other device – actual paper really helps you think clearly) and come up with a physical list. It could be cooking your favourite meal. It could be doing yoga. It could be having sex. It could be turning up your favourite song really loud and jumping around like a lunatic. It could be lighting your treasured Diptyque and sinking into a bath with a face mask on.

Once you are out of the cycle of over-drinking to numb stress you will feel so much better in so many ways. Not only will you feel calmer, happier and have more energy, you will also look better, which is always a confidence boost. However, it would be naive to think that, once you're in control of your drinking, you'll never have a bad day. Life still happens, and it can still be shit. What you have to do is be prepared. If you stick to your alternative treats most of the time, that well-deserved occasional G&T will taste all the more special.

DRINK-FREE DISTRACTIONS

- Make a playlist of tracks to lift your mood. Don't try to be cool, choose what genuinely makes you want to dance. I won't judge (as long as you don't judge my love of Carly Rae Jepsen).
- Watch a YouTube tutorial of something that you've always wanted to learn. It could be anything from doing a French braid to bleeding a radiator.
- Sign up for a kick-ass exercise class. Something like boxing is a great way to vent work stress.
- Watch a TED talk. I'd recommend Brené Brown's presentation on the power of vulnerability, Elizabeth Gilbert on harnessing your elusive creative genius, or Steve Jobs on how to live before you die.

WRITE YOUR DRINK-FREE DISTRACTIONS HERE

....
....
....
....
....
....
....
....
....
....
....
....
....
....
....
....
....
....
....
....
....
....
....
....
....
....

TRICK YOUR BRAIN

Do you keep beers in the fridge, just in case? Are your wine glasses arranged on an exposed shelf? You might even have a rather lovely old-school drinks trolley, full of bottles of spirits. Displaying booze paraphernalia, and having drinks available in case anyone pops round, feels like part of being a grown-up. It's the same as having a coffee machine, or some nice mugs. But these things can be your downfall (not the coffee machine, unless you are also cutting back on caffeine right now, to which I would say, hold your horses, let's do one thing at a time).

The availability of alcohol in our immediate physical surroundings is incredibly important. It sounds ridiculous that keeping red wine in the cupboard, rather than out on your kitchen shelf, would make any difference at all to how much you drink. But studies have shown that it does. Ideally, don't have alcohol in the house at all and, if you don't find it too weird, change into your pyjamas as soon as you get home from work. It just makes going out to buy wine that bit more inconvenient.

One American study from 2014[28] identified simple tricks that can make you drink less without even realising it. Participants in the study poured 12 per cent more wine when they had a wider glass, compared to a narrower one. So ditch those stylish-looking

28 A study in the *International Journal of Drug Policy*, conducted by researchers at Iowa State and Cornell Universities

coupe glasses for your fizz and stick to a traditional flute. When all other elements were the same, subjects poured 9 per cent more white wine than they did red, which researchers put down to the greater colour contrast of dark wine in a clear glass making it appear more full. And, perhaps most surprisingly, holding the glass in your hand as it's being filled up resulted in a 12 per cent bigger serving than if the wine was poured into a glass on a table.

The most important thing that the study uncovered, however, was the simple trick of only pouring yourself half a glass of wine at a time. Participants were told they could drink as much as they like, but the only caveat was they must only half-fill each glass. In doing this, female subjects drank 27 per cent less than the women who were allowed to pour a full glass each time. The men drank 26 per cent less. You can't get a much easier strategy than that, and it's a particularly good one for drinking at home. Just tell yourself you can have as much wine as you want, only half a glass at a time. You'll realise that you've had enough far sooner.

People tend to think of drinks in terms of 'a drink'. So they'll say they had three glasses of wine, regardless of whether they were small or large glasses. The obvious solution here is always go for the smaller option. Always. Just make that a standard rule. A small glass of wine and a single-measure spirit will give you just as much enjoyment as the larger version.

If you're thinking right now that these tips are ridiculous, and there's no way you will drink less simply because you only have half a glass at a time, that's totally normal. The power of these techniques is in the fact that every single person thinks they're immune to them. But none of us are. And, left to its own devices, your mind will play tricks of its own: making you feel like you're missing out because you didn't have a drink, or as if you failed because you did have one. You now know how many impulses, decisions and judgements come from your unconscious mind, rather than from any logical place, so you might as well make that mind work for you.

TRICK-YOUR-BRAIN CHECKLIST

- Don't keep alcohol at home. Or if you must, keep it out of sight.
- Make it as inconvenient as possible to pop out and buy wine.
- Drink from the smallest, narrowest glass you can find.
- Only pour half a glass at a time.
- Always order a small glass of wine, or a single measure of spirits.

TRY THIS

Ignore those supermarket special offers. Yes, it's cheaper to buy six bottles of wine, but you only need one for that dinner party. Don't just add it to your order saying, 'it'll get drunk eventually', because we all know that 'eventually' will end up being before the end of next week.

....

A NOTE ON MINDFUL EATING

Since there is a huge amount of sugar in most alcoholic drinks (unless you're knocking back straight vodka, in which case the sugar content is the least of your concerns), many people find that cutting down on drinking increases their sweet tooth. Perhaps you've never really been a dessert person before, but now that chocolate pudding on the menu is calling to you. Normally you just pick up a coffee in the morning, but now you're looking at that blueberry muffin in a new light. This is totally normal, and is something to which your body will acclimatise as you get used to drinking less. The good news is that many of the mindfulness techniques you have learnt throughout this book in relation to alcohol can be used with food, too. Do you really need that chocolate biscuit? Is the real issue stress, loneliness or boredom? Can you surf the urge?

You can deal with this in the same way that you have dealt with drinking; don't let it build up in your mind and become a massive issue that makes you want to over-drink again.

'People worry about the fact that they suddenly wake up in a Haribo coma,' says Laura Willoughby, 'but it is natural that you crave sweet things or putting things in your mouth after changing your drinking. If people start to worry that drinking less is making them eat shit, then that brings in the failure mentality. Instead, they should give themselves a little bit of a break and focus on the main thing, and see healthy eating as a side product. They are aligned goals. Other healthy habits will support your change in drinking.'

Long term, drinking less is only going to make you thinner. Not only because you are no longer consuming the mountains of sugar and calories in drinks, but also you'll have fewer junk-food cravings and energy crashes, leading to you wanting something sweet or carby. You will be less likely to reach for an unhealthy snack, and you can enjoy an all-round greater sense of awareness and control about what you're putting into your body. This is the start of a healthier relationship with food as much as it is with booze.

TRY THIS

Don't get involved in rounds in the pub. Ever knocked back the second half of your drink in one gulp because you realised someone else has finished and it's your round? Setting up a tab, to be split at the end of the night, is a better option.

YOUR INNER CIRCLE

Drinking has probably always been a big part of your social life. Perhaps one of your friends is the type of person who doesn't think an evening is fun unless they have no memory of the latter part of it. You know, the kind of person who would describe themselves as a 'legend'. Or perhaps you were that person, and your friends are having trouble getting used to the new you.

Your friends and family may even get quite defensive when you tell them that you're not drinking, or drinking less. This doesn't happen with anything else. For instance, I don't like mushrooms, but when I turn down something with mushrooms in it, I'm not confronted with a barrage of opinions about how boring it is to not have mushrooms, or how this mushroom is a particularly good vintage, or I should have a mushroom because it's so-and-so's birthday.

Sadly, it's often those closest to us who are most likely to sabotage us, and they'll do so in the name of generosity or hospitality. Proponents of Alcoholics Anonymous's 12-Step programme call this 'enabling', and it happens all the time. I recently saw a post on Instagram from a woman who was trying to drink less and, struggling with cravings; she was asking for advice. 'Life is short,' read a comment underneath, 'drink the wine'. With what other substance would people so casually and dismissively try to undermine your good intentions? This is where you must be very strong and not give in to feeling obliged to drink.

They say that you become the five people you spend the most time with. So, while you interact with many people, it's the handful you see most often that shape who you are. People's values, behaviours and attitudes inevitably rub off on those around them. Think about that. Who are the five people you spend most time with? Do you want to be like them? You can't do much about an irritating colleague or family member, but there are plenty of opportunities elsewhere in your life to surround yourself with the kind of people that inspire you to be the best version of yourself.

Take a break from your heaviest-drinking friends, just for now, while you're getting the hang of your new relationship with alcohol. Or try to meet them during the day for lunch or coffee, or go to the cinema. Remember to always be actively kind – to yourself, as well as to others. Don't blame them for trying to make you drink. And don't blame yourself if you make the choice not to have them around for a while.

There may be a person in your life who is negative and drinks too much, but that person is a long-standing friend and, despite (or perhaps because of) their issues, you don't feel that you can simply ditch them. That's admirable, but don't let it become a toxic relationship in which you allow yourself to be coerced into drinking simply to make them feel better. Long term, you know it's not going to make them feel better anyway.

Being more aware of your own thoughts – as you now are, thanks to the mindfulness techniques – will help you be kinder towards other people. Practise patience and understanding. If a person wants you to drink because they are, that isn't your problem: it's entirely theirs. But it is possible to move through that situation without making them feel like you are judging them for drinking.

Your partner can be an unlikely stumbling block. My husband and I used to share a bottle of wine pretty much every night. When I was pregnant, he switched to beer (out of solidarity because, since I'm not a beer drinker, I didn't covet his beer as I would have a glass of wine). This habit has stuck, and he still drinks beer almost every night. I'd rather he didn't – not least because he's a beer snob who only drinks those craft ales that cost an arm and a leg – but I have to concede that it's his decision.

Sharing with people what you're doing will help strengthen your commitment, but think carefully about who you disclose this to. Perhaps telling your heavy drinking friend will only make them feel bad about themselves and they may try to talk you out of it, or undermine your determination. Once you have identified a supportive friend – perhaps one who already drinks moderately, or wants to do so – tell them, and make sure they know how important their cheerleading is, and how grateful you are for it.

Your relationships are key to your happiness, and social cohesion is vital for reducing anxiety, so don't hide away from the world because you have decided to drink less. Never feel that you can't go to the pub with friends. Drinking alcohol in the pub is not compulsory.

If you're struggling to get your friends on board, find a community online. Club Soda has everything from a very active (private) Facebook group to regular meet-ups and events nationwide.

'Whether you're moderating or going alcohol-free, being social is one of the most important things,' agrees Laura Willoughby. 'We use University College London's behaviour change taxonomy, and one of the biggest is that being social is the superfood of behaviour change. If you can find other people on the same journey, or if you can find ways to be social, then the chances of being able to change are greater. That's why we do our lunches so that people, regardless of their goal, can come and have an alcohol-free lunch. They feel a lot more comfortable because they have people to talk to about their not drinking.'

Having said that, the chances are that if you feel like you want to cut down, some of your friends probably do too. It's true that you can't change anyone else's behaviour, only your own, but once they see you with bright eyes and radiant skin, living a life free from hangxiety, feeling happier and healthier than ever before, I bet they will want to moderate their own drinking, too.

TRY THIS

Now that you're drinking less, make it count. Forty per cent of global alcohol brands are controlled by just ten companies. Buying from smaller producers gives you the smug glow of knowing you are supporting a friendly local gin distiller or craft brewery, which is significantly nicer than giving your cash to some huge conglomerate.

....

NOTES

5

RELAPSE

It happens. The key to getting over this is simply to accept it for what it is, continue to believe that you're on the right path and put it behind you.

It's easy to fall into the trap of feeling that, since you 'failed' at your moderate drinking goal last night, you must have some kind of problem. There's that pesky inner dialogue again: 'I've tried, but I can't stop. Alcohol has power over me.' This leads to a depressing vicious circle of attempting to abstain, failing, then feeling difficult emotions such as frustration, guilt, regret, shame, anger and our old friend anxiety. These feelings can all be triggers for drinking. Knock that process on the head by acknowledging them. Rohan Gunatillake calls them 'inner monsters', and he makes a case for addressing them directly.

'When you have challenging thoughts rampaging through your mind, try naming them and saying hello,' he writes in *Modern Mindfulness: How to Be More Relaxed, Focused, and Kind While Living in a Fast, Digital, Always-On World*. '"Hello anxiety. Hello guilt. Why, hello there Mr Sense-Of-Feeling-Worthless. So lovely to see you again!" Doing this can not only externalise the experience but it can also puncture its power due to the lightness of it all. To add even more effectiveness, say hello to those monsters aloud if you can. Once you've named them you will be much quicker at noticing when they come back.'

Once you've acknowledged your feelings about relapsing, take the opportunity to reflect on what it was that triggered you to drink more than you wanted to. Go as far back in the process as you can. Perhaps you think you agreed to a drink after work because your willpower was weak today, but when you look back, could that argument you had with your partner in the morning have had anything to do with it? What about that passive-aggressive email from your boss? Were you feeling angry or vulnerable? Acknowledge those feelings to get to the root of them. Yes, this takes vigilance, which initially seems like a lot of effort, but with practice and repetition it will quickly become second nature.

The most important thing about this process is that you carry it out with with compassion and forgiveness, as you would if you were talking to a close friend about the same thing.

Think about how you might behave differently when the same set of circumstances conspires against you in the future (and you know it will). Then recommit to your plan by looking at your list of Mindful Drinking Motivation again.

Ruby Warrington doesn't like to call falling off the wagon a 'relapse', she calls it a 'reminder'. Think of it as meeting up with an old flame – a person you always looked back on with rose-tinted spectacles, remembering the great sex and forgetting all about the selfishness, the laziness and the moodiness. After an hour in his company, you know that you made the right decision in ending that particular relationship.

Learn to see a relapse as something positive, because it's an opportunity for you to see with clarity the feelings, situations or people that might trigger you to drink too much. And once you've recognised that, it makes the rest of your journey easier. As you read this book and contemplate your journey of moderation, there will be constant small shifts in your perception about how much you need alcohol in your life. These changes are almost imperceptible, but they add up to a reinvention.

Another reason why you might stumble is that positive change might not feel immediately apparent for everyone. Perhaps, initially, without alcohol to numb your anxieties, you're actually feeling more stressed out and less able to sleep, and perhaps you're eating crap food as a substitute, or you're finding sober socialising a struggle. Ultimately, all of these things will be vastly improved by drinking less, but in the early days of habit change it's perfectly normal to feel discombobulated. Do not let it throw you off track.

Yes, moderation takes commitment, but it's commitment to something that will make your life significantly better. When you marry the man of your dreams, you don't waste any time thinking about all the losers you can no longer sleep with. Not having that hastily guzzled cheap white wine in your life is no loss.

Laura Willoughby recommends establishing daily modera-tion practice. 'What we find really useful at Club Soda is immers-ing yourself in the topic,' she says. 'Put time aside every day to put some practice into your not drinking. Maybe that's reading a blog, reading through some top tips, talking to a community, getting some advice for your alcohol-free days ... Nearly all the tools for going alcohol-free are the same for when you're moder-ating. Changing your drinking is a practice.'

And remember to keep practising sober socialising and sober stress-relievers. Like anything in life, the more you practise, the better you'll get. Social support is vital, so rope in some friends or sign up for an online community, such as joinclubsoda.co.uk or thisnakedmindcommunity.com.

'Community is so important,' says Annie Grace, author of *This Naked Mind.* 'We are motivated by other people's stories. We are social beings; in fact, it is of evolutionary importance that we are motivated to be part of a tribe. We function better when we have the support of others.'

If you feel you need more help, try a meditation course, or try hypnotherapy. Give yourself the best possible chance, because once you have established your more moderate lifestyle, you will find that it is no longer a daily struggle.

Annie Grace tells me she believes a moderate relationship with alcohol is absolutely possible, 'as long as the drinker exer-cises mindfulness, and is well-educated and cautious. 'There are certainly pitfalls to moderate drinking, because alcohol creates a thirst for itself, but I truly do think it is an individual journey and promoting complete abstinence as the only way forward (when it is not necessary for many people) makes questioning our drinking scarier than it should be.'

Your own journey of moderation might take several attempts. And you might spend a lot of time weighing up whether your fear of Sunday morning 'hangxiety' is greater or lesser than your fear of sober socialising. If you're wavering, go back to your Mindful Drinking Motivation list and remind yourself why you're doing this.

You *can* find freedom from alcohol. Just be kind to yourself, and remember: alcohol does not control you any more. You control it.

NOTES

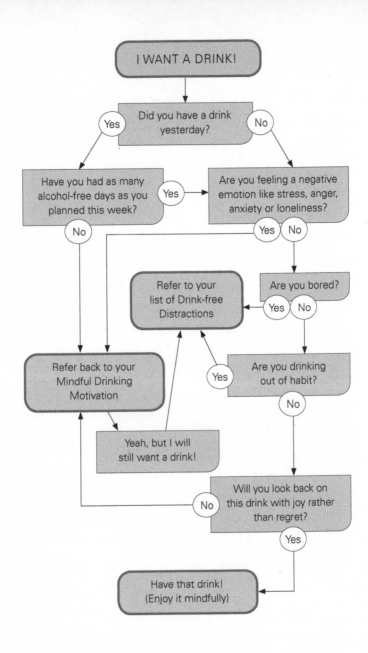

CONCLUSION

By now you have assessed your drinking behaviour and completed a 28-day Clean Break. You have set goals and committed to your own personal rules. You've learned to look at the underlying reasons why you drink in order to identify your triggers, and you've planned for any pitfalls you might encounter, including your friends and family. You have adopted tools such as monitoring, reflection, distraction, reframing, visualisation and gratitude, and you've braved sober socialising. You have learned to live more mindfully, too, in a way that works for you. And after 12 weeks you will check in again for your evaluation and not beat yourself up about any relapses you might have had. These techniques changed my life, and they can change yours, too.

You've got this far, and you now know that you do not *need* alcohol. You are the same person with a lime and soda in your hand as you are with a gin and tonic, but you're also sharper, smarter, slimmer, healthier and glowing from the inside. You're kinder and more thoughtful, too, because you're more conscious of what is going on around you and aware of how other people are feeling.

I like the person I am when I drink less, in fact I like that person way more than the slurring, stumbling party girl who, let's face it, was actually significantly less fun than I thought I was at the time.

The empowering effect of your new lifestyle grows the more you do it. The more alcohol-free days you have, and the more times you attend and get through an event alcohol-free at which you previously couldn't have imagined not drinking: those things will make you feel stronger by proving you can do it, and reinforcing that positive message in your unconscious mind.

Please do let me know how you get on – you can find me on Twitter or Instagram @RosamundDean – because I want to hear your success stories, as well as your slip-ups. Hey, we *all* have them.

Mindful drinking is *not* about deprivation; it's about freedom. So enjoy this process, as much as you enjoy reaping the benefits of it.

Make the effort to memorise these five points below – etch them indelibly onto your brain, setting good intentions for life – and feel galvanised and empowered to continue drinking moderately forever.

Preparation is everything. Always have a plan for when you intend to drink, and how much. Never make an exception on the spur of the moment.

Don't use alcohol to deal with difficult or stressful situations, such as family dramas or office politics. Tempting as it may be, it *never* makes a situation better.

Let go of perfection. If you get wasted and wake up feeling terrible, do not feel that now you might as well have a Bloody Mary with brunch. Learn from the relapse instead and set new intentions.

Be present. In everything you do – that will help you stop that craving for wine in its tracks, as well as ensure you fully enjoy it when you do decide to drink.

You. Can. Do. This. Remember, anxiety leads to drinking, which leads to anxiety, and so it goes on. Once you start drinking mindfully and you realise you *can* do sober socialising, your confidence and happiness levels will increase. As will your energy and productivity. Although it might be hard at first, with repetition your good habits will stick. And the better you feel, the less you will need to drink. Have you heard of a 'virtuous circle'? It's the opposite of a vicious circle and you're in one right now. I'll say cheers to that.

REFERENCES

Club Soda: joinclubsoda.co.uk

DrinkAware: www.drinkaware.co.uk

Seedlip: www.seedlipdrinks.com

Shrb: www.shrbdrinks.com

Andy Cope, *Happiness: Your Route-Map to Inner Joy*, John Murray Learning (2017)

Annie Grace, *This Naked Mind: Control Alcohol: Find Freedom, Rediscover Happiness & Change Your Life*, ASPN Publications (2015)

Rohan Gunatillake, *Modern Mindfulness: How to Be More Relaxed, Focused, and Kind While Living in a Fast, Digital, Always-On World*, Bluebird (2017)

Victoria Moore, *The Wine Dine Dictionary: Good Food and Good Wine: An A-Z of Suggestions for Happy Eating and Drinking*, Granta (2017)

Eleanor Morgan, *Anxiety for Beginners: A Personal Investigation*, Bluebird (2016)

Gretchen Rubin, *The Four Tendencies: The Indispensable Personality Profiles That Reveal How to Make Your Life Better (and Other People's Lives Better, Too)*, Two Roads (2017)

Shona Vertue, *The Vertue Method: A stronger, fitter, healthier you – in 28 days*, Yellow Kite (2017)

Ruby Warrington, *Material Girl, Mystical World: The Now-Age Guide for Chic Seekers and Modern Mystics*, HarperCollins (2017)

ACKNOWLEDGEMENTS

Thank you to my agent, Chris Wellbelove, for being the architect of everything. And to my editor, Sam Eades, who laughed it off when, the first time we met, I accidentally knocked my glass of rosé all over her. How times have changed.

Sam's clear vision and razor-sharp judgement, and Anna Valentine's astute edits, were indispensable. I'm so happy to be part of the Trapeze family of bold, brilliant books.

Thank you to Debbie Holmes and Helen Ewing for creating the beautiful cover, Helena Caldon for lightning-fast copy editing, Elizabeth Allen for publicity prowess, Katie Horrocks for production wizardry and Paul Stark in the audio team, for letting me read my own audiobook.

I met and interviewed many experts over the course of my research, but would particularly like to thank Laura Willoughby MBE and Dr Jussi Tolvi of Club Soda, and Rohan Gunatillake of buddhify. They are pioneers in helping people live better in a way that is both aspirational and accessible.

Thank you to Sarah Bailey, my editor at Red, for her support and encouragement, and Red's wellness guru Brigid Moss, for first sending me off to be hypnotised into drinking less, and for her wise advice.

I'm grateful to my children, Ezra and Eden, for making me want to drink less. But I couldn't have written this book without some kind people taking them off my hands, so thank you to my mother-in-law, Anne, and my mum, Hélène.

And, most importantly, thank you to my husband Jonathan, who did some exceptional solo parenting (admittedly often in the pub) while I wrote, then talked me calmly through edits and restored my confidence during deadline-related hysteria. I don't know where I'd be without him. Probably still drunk.